T0367528

Mr. Rhoads is the author of a series of Self-Health books: "Never Too Old to Live", "The Boomers Are Coming", "Remedy Eldercide", "Restore Elder Pride", "American Enterprise Manifesto", "America In The Red Zone".

Also upcoming books: "THE BIGGEST BULLY (In The China Shop)" and "How to Win the Monopsony Game".

He and his wife are in their mid-seventies and are living examples of what the Self-Health movement is all about . . . family, healthy habits and a love for each other. In Part I of the Book the impact of better habits is the primary topic and in Part II the mental conditioning exercises for forming better habits is the impetus to changing the mind's focus from unhealthy thoughts to positive Self-Health results.

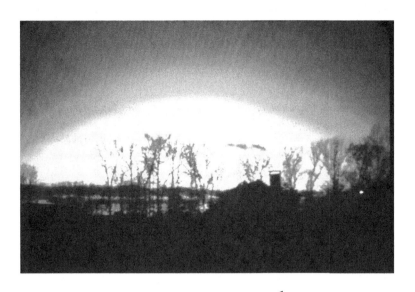

America in the
Red Zone

In Pursuit of the Self-Health End Zone Diet

A Self-Health Book

JERRY RHOADS

iUniverse LLC
Bloomington

AMERICA IN THE RED ZONE
IN PURSUIT OF THE SELF-HEALTH END ZONE DIET

iUniverse books may be ordered through booksellers or by contacting:

iUniverse LLC
1663 Liberty Drive
Bloomington, IN 47403
www.iuniverse.com
1-800-Authors (1-800-288-4677)

ISBN: 978-1-4917-1946-6 (sc)
ISBN: 978-1-4917-1948-0 (hc)
ISBN: 978-1-4917-1947-3 (e)

Library of Congress Control Number: 2014900200

Printed in the United States of America.

iUniverse rev. date: 03/03/2014

TABLE OF CONTENTS

PART I
Red Zone Habits In Pursuit of
the Self-Health End Zone

PART II
Red Zone Thinking in Pursuit of
The Self-Health End Zone

PREFACE

Health Care Lost

Paradise Lost, Wars Lost, Hope Lost, Businesses Lost, Homeland Lost, Health Care Lost. The Cost of Restoring Health in America is lost on most people because they don't have to pay the bills. Medicare, Medicaid, Insurance, Veterans, free care for the indigent, etc. step up and pay for illness with wellness being lost in the pursuit of money. Economists call this the externalism syndrome . . . when it doesn't cost us personally it is external to our values.

America is in the Red Zone of health meaning the bad habits of prior life styles are catching up with more and more overweight, chronically ill patients either in recovery from chemical dependency or food dependency. 77 million Americans are reaching retirement age this decade with many maladies that result in needing health care services. 10,000 per week are signing up for Medicare and there is Obama Care saying the Government enforces will cut $500 billion out of the program in the next 10 years.

BABY BOOMERS BY JERRY RHOADS

The Boomers are coming
The impact is stunning
After the end of the Great war in '45
Brides and Grooms came alive

Boosting the pregnancy rate
Opening the baby gate
Christening 77 million by '65
Putting us in economic overdrive

Starting in 2005 they want to retire
Long before they expire
Maxing out their social security checks
Leaving entitlements as fiscal wrecks

Paying their share of tax bills if wealthy
Believing that Medicare will keep them healthy
Being the driving force of the Great Society
What they were promised is impropriety

However like much in today's politics
The Boomers will demand and vote for a fix
Finding no equity in money-tics
Like the ride of Paul Revere

"Never fear The Boomers are here"

The following chart shows the number of U.S. births from 1946 to 1994 in total births:

Year	Total Births
1946	3,400,000
1947	3,800,000
1948	3,600,000
1949	3,600,000
1950	3,600,000
1951	3,600,000
1952	3,800,000
1953	3,800,000
1954	4,100,000
1955	4,100,000
1956	4,200,000
1957	4,200,000
1958	4,200,000
1959	4,200,000
1960	4,200,000
1961	4,250,000
1962	4,250,000
1963	4,100,000
1964	4,100,000
Total	77,000,000

After American soldiers returned home from World War II. the United States experienced an "explosion" of births.

The Baby Boomer Generation is generally defined as those born between the years of 1946 and 1964.

Let's see how that breaks down:
per year: 4,000,000
per day (4.0 mil / 365): 10,958
per hour (10.6 k / 24): 456
per minute (456 / 60): 7.1

And 7.1 per minute amounts to one every 8.5 seconds.

Along with the changing nature of the health care clientele are certain realities facing each every State. Medicaid will be the safety net for those under the poverty level and health care exchanges are envisioned by the bureaucrats to pick up the rest of the population. So the States are being prompted by Obama's plan to enact Self-Health initiatives and become the healthiest State in the Union. The Self-Health movement is a not for profit venture started by **the best-selling book The Blue Zones where the author and explorer Dan Buettner chronicles the "Lessons for Living Longer from the People Who've Lived the Longest who w**ith the right lifestyle, experts say, may live up to a decade longer. Since the Red Zone Baby Boomers are coming at us at the unrelenting speed of 7,000 per week into a health care system that cannot handle the three million currently needing health care services a shift in the paradigm to a (SHIFT) Self-Health Insurance Funding Trust is inevitable (see www.singaporehealthcare.com for a self-funding program being used more successfully than America's Obama Care will ever be). The Singapore solution and my proposed SHIFT program puts the responsibility for improved health care habits internalized to each individual and that in itself cuts illness costs and improves wellness outcomes.

The cost of illness escalation is eating up national resources faster than we can cover them. The average cost of an outpatient procedure in a hospital is more than $15,000 . . . inpatient $100,000 . . . a month's stay in a skilled nursing home $7,000 . . . a year over $60,000 . . . a monthly stay in assisted living $6,000 . . . cost per hour for accountants servicing health care $300 per hour . . . attorneys $500 per hour and malpractice claims in the millions . . . Hospice care $700 per day . . . Home care $1,000 per day . . . when is it going to stop!

At the same time Society is gaining weight at an astounding rate, there are over 2.5 million falls per year for aging Americans, there are 8 billion pills passed to aging Americans in nursing homes, there is $50 billion dollars per year spent on enforcing and avoiding the intrusion of Government regulations, there are $1 trillion in Obama Care for the extrusion of funding for academic demonstration projects over the next 10 years to supposedly improve quality of care and life of the aging Americans and another $1 trillion dollars in the next 10 years for enforcement of that Affordable Health Care Act by the IRS.

According to studies there are not enough primary care physicians now let alone the 12 multiple looking us in the face for doctors, nurses, therapists over the next 10 years to treat escalating illnesses. The Government in all there lack of vision has restrained the development of nursing home beds for the last 20 years with plans of keeping the sickly elderly at home with relatives. Bleak as it seems these problems need solutions or we will all be at home taking care of the sick and dependent relatives. Instead of academic testing we need entrepreneurial outcomes creating savings.

1. Self-Health programs for preventing chronic illnesses, obesity and depression.
2. Reduction of chemicals ingested by Americans.
3. Physical and mental exercising that fights off obesity and depression.
4. Health preservation initiatives by health and fitness experts.
5. De-institutionalization of the elderly and disabled.
6. Natural health remedies promoted and provided by health professionals.
7. Most importantly resources used to pay for outcomes not incomes . . . define outcomes as the reduction of known

health and illness problems . . . not just symptomatic guesses or medical diagnosis without root cause analysis.

8. Replace inductive pursuit of treatment to deductive pursuit of cause and effect.
9. Get Government out of the health care business and eliminate 60% of the wasted resources.
10. Elect government officials that have knowledge and expertise in Health Care delivery and funding.

America currently expends $2.4 trillion dollars on poor health, pills and treatment . . . we pay more for illness than wellness. Obama Care further monetizes (pays for) illness without any practical solutions for paying for the pursuit of outcomes (cures, prevention of chronic diseases, fitness or wellness activities). Capitation (where payment is for groups of individuals in a high or low risk pool without consideration of individual needs and services) reimbursement and managed care population methods are only focused on service reduction not efficiency and effective quality controls. This approach is forecasted to cost $1.1 trillion and generate $1.2 trillion in provider taxes over the next decade.

This is the most serious wasteful problem we have . . . so our focus should be on common scientific knowledge not on wishful programs out of political academia (universities with grants and bureaucratic think tanks). By truly paying for outcomes (results) not incomes (money for treatment, tests and drugs with no known benefit) we begin to construct meaningful Enterprise payment for performance managed by the private sector. Doing away with enforcement rules and regulations based on illness that do not pay for improved health or wellness. The pursuit of wellness for the Baby Boomers will save trillions that are now being wasted on hospital ER, tests, treatment, physician prescriptions, nursing home illnesses, home care sickness and hospice end of life comfort costs.

Jerry Rhoads the author is a CPA and Fellow in the American College of health Care Administrators, licensed in many States and a recognized expert on Medicare and Medicaid payment programs and has been involved in health care since 1962 as an accountant, consultant, systems designer, operator, government advisor plus having written hundreds of articles, manuals, books on the subject. His latest books, including this one, are a series of Self-Health books (**Remedy Eldercide, iUniverse; Restore Elder Pride, iUniverse; Never Too Old to Live, Xlibris; and The Boomers are Coming, (SHIFT the Paradigm to Self-Health), Xlibris**) that propose shifting the paradigm to individual self-health plans funded by withholding accounts to remove the waste out of the current system. It is proposed to take the funding out of the wasteful Government run Obama Care to private sector Mutual Health Insurance Companies owned by its policy holders that would process Health Preservation claims. $600 billion per year can be saved changing the method of payment from treatment and drugs to outcome and prevention. We then get something for money invested in Enterprise Health Care organizations that are accountable to their shareholders (policy holders). In the author's context we move the Red Zone pursuit of treatment and medications to a more Self-Health science driven deductive process where the clinical professionals are using natural remedies, technology and data to perform services based on more natural diagnostic testing to preserve health and prevent disease rather than accept that least invasive procedures and interventions used to rule out what they cannot inductively prove. We then can have incentive Health Science managing the Restorative Model deductively and profitably, rather than the Government inductive Medical Model in an art form using enforcement and fear as the control method.

THE END ZONE THINKING DIET
by Jerry Rhoads

The thinking person's diet
You need to try it
It is not deprivation
More like motivation
Schooled in doubt
Americans think you must go without
But to be the perfect size and weight
One needs to be happier about one's fate
Because in reality all it is
Is change one's thinking to show biz
Being beautiful is made up
And image is not to be fed up
It is what the mind decides
With some help from your insides
Telling you what to do and what to eat
Overcoming fear that we have to defeat
Ourselves to win
When stinking thinking is our only sin
Say the following phrase to start you days
To make yourself the brunt of praise
"I am who I am, to be what I can
According to my Self-Health End Zone thinking plan"

INTRODUCTION

Shifting The Paradigm: From Red Zone Habits to Self-Health End Zone Thinking

Self-Health is defined as each individual accepting responsibility for their own decisions that affect their health care costs. A Funding trust through withholding from employees' salaries and allowing them to spend the funds on preventive health measures and preservation of their own future health care needs, reduces expenditures for the Greater Good 40% and improves outcomes 100%.

The national problem is that 80% of the $2.2 trillion spent on illness is in the last 2 years of people's lives. This does not meet the health needs of the rest of the Americans. It is reactive not preventive in its infrastructure. There is $400 to $600 billion in waste in the system. To Grow the economy . . . create jobs and encourage expansion of the Health services, as the largest service provider in the world, the waste must be eliminated and the savings better spent on improving wellness, prevention of illness and preservation of health. This new Health Service industry can cut costs and improve American's health. The systemic solution is as follows:

1) Computerized self-assessment of health condition required for each American annually for the purpose of establishing

health care rates for the SHIFT (self-health insurance funding trust) program.

2) National data base created for analysis of health problems and setting rates to be used by physicians to diagnose, prevent and treat illnesses, especially chronic diseases.

3) Wellness plan printed for each American's problems and transported with the patient before utilizing health care services, except for emergency services.

4) Over medication and re-hospitalization of the elderly must be reduced and eradicated as much as possible.

Health service companies will have to base their services on each individual's health-fitness profile using computer models of care with anticipated outcomes for individualized problems. Each service provider would be paid on an economic incentive formula for improving wellness and each American would pay premiums based on their Self-Health profile.

Serving The Greater Good— Through An Enterprise Model

The foundation of American democracy is the pursuit of the greater good. As a country, we pursue what is good for most of the people, most of the time. But that is not our approach for the care of our elderly. Of the 313 million people in America, 77 million are baby boomers. In the next ten years, a staggering majority of them will turn sixty. Even though it would be for the greater good of America, there are no provisions for taking care of these aging lives.

There are only time bombs:

- Currently, there are 3.2 million falls per year among the elderly in nursing homes. There will be 80 million per year when the baby boomers come of nursing home age.

- On the average, baby boomers will have four to five chronic illnesses by the time they are sixty-five, that equates to 350 million chronic conditions.
- Seventy-seven million families will be affected by the disabilities and chronic conditions imposed on them by aging baby boomers.
- Seventy-seven million households are not equipped and never will be to handle chronic illnesses and dependent lives.
- About $77 trillion will be imposed annually on the budgets of state and federal governments to care for the aging boomers.
- Seventy-seven million voters will be enraged by the lack of preparation for and health care coverage for the greater good.
- Those same 77 million voters, with an average yearly spending of 50K that adds up to $3.86 trillion, do NOT want to spend their money on the current health care system. They would rather invest in health preservation than in health maintenance.
- The 46 million uninsured will become 100 million as the baby boomers become of retirement age and unemployed.
- There are currently 1.7 million nursing home patients in 16,000 nursing homes and 4 million assisted—living residents in 23,000 assisted-living facilities. We will need seventeen times as many nursing homes and eighteen times as many assisted-living facilities to handle the 77 million baby boomers in a supportive setting.
- One million physicians, 2.4 million nurses, 4,500 hospitals, 16,000 nursing homes and 6.4 million other health professionals cannot handle the needs of 77 million aging baby boomers who want their share of the health care dollars. Making the radical change from health maintenance to prevention and health preservation would serve the greater good and make more Medicare money available.

On top of these time bombs, we have 77 million high expectations. If we are expecting these 77 million baby boomers to just accept nursing homes and assisted living as they are, think again. They tend to be dependent on others for their approach to health care and generally are not staying healthy; nor are they schooled in preserving their health and do not want to pay more for preventing poor health. Compounding this, their health care providers are not schooled in detecting cause or in pursuing measurable outcomes. But they are paid regardless of results.

For example: I have a relative who is a baby boomer, and she has a sinus problem that has been going on for over a year. During that time, her ear, nose and throat specialist had her on four different antibiotics to treat a bacterial infection (one of which caused her to lose excessive weight), then performed a $28,000 sinus surgery that turned into a life-threatening episode due to mismanagement of her recovery, then three different nasal solutions to treat a so-called viral infection, then on an antifungal solution to treat a now-diagnosed fungus; and she still has the infection, and still no one knows what caused it nor what will cure it. In the meantime, everyone gets paid, and she continues to suffer. Then after all this a cardiologist diagnosed her with congestive heart disease not sinus infection . . . she had a pace maker installed and has not had problems since.

AN ENTERPRISE MODEL

What we need for the greater good is not more rhetoric. The words reform, transform, fine-tune, and incrementally change are not going to meet the needs of the greater good. The health care paradigm must **SHIFT (self-health** insurance funding trusts) to the following four postulates:

1. Switch from a system of health maintenance or disease management to one of health preservation. The greater good will be served if the 77 million baby boomers are

focused on preserving wellness through fitness, nutrition, social relationships, and prevention instead of reacting to and treating illness. Then the focus can be on the following funding principles for our future health care system:

a. Embrace a National Health Policy for Universal Health Insurance funded by an individual withholding concept with personal savings accounts and tax deductions for health preservation investments.

b. Take the employers out of the middle and assign the cost of poor health habits to the individual savings accounts funded by a mandatory withholding program similar to the Medicare withholding program.

c. Vote for a comprehensive change in the way current services are paid for (pay for outcomes: reduction of medications, prevention of re-hospitalization, and screenings, not just testing for treatment).

  i. Provide the economic incentives to providers for profiting from wellness and preventing illness so the greater good can be attained.

  ii. Pay the providers of future health care services for preservation outcomes: restoring health, preventing chronic diseases, and preserving wellness.

d. Pay for the uninsured and underinsured out of the cost savings by eliminating the waste in the current system by these four postulates.

2. Eliminate the acceptance of chronic disease as the responsibility of the health care providers or the employers of America. Support and reward the 77 million baby boomers for embracing wellness as a lifestyle regardless of age.

3. Educate the physicians, nurses, therapists, social workers, etc., to use care planning for the pursuit of outcomes.

4. Train the health professionals to use technology for diagnosing the cause of disease, preventing reoccurrences, preserving wellness, and treating illnesses.

Preventative care and health preservation services not only serve the greater good but also would be cheaper in the long run. The radical shift necessary to pursue prevention and health preservation, instead of treatment, may not be the first choice of America's five million health care professionals. It may not be the first choice of the 16,000 nursing home operators. But it should be America's first choice because it will serve the greater good. It will better serve the lives of the 77 million baby boomers and the 6 million people in nursing homes and assisted care. All Americans have the right to stay healthy, for the greater good.

My mother and father were old when they were in their forties, characterized by their use of false teeth, thoughts of early retirement, being out of shape, being in poor health, and destined to be in a nursing home living out their final years in miserable conditions. They were both victims of Eldercide or the systematic institutionalization of the elderly after a chronic illness.

I, at the age of seventy-four, on the other hand, have all my teeth; think in terms of late retirement; am taking no medications; have less than 10% body fat; destined to avoid institutional confinement for as long as humanly possible. Having my own business with my wife and son as partners is the motivation for my most productive life beginning at seventy, together with my three daughters who all are career businesswomen and looking forward to late retirement. My wife, also has all her teeth, beautiful hair, enviable figure, and a no Botox face who wants to stay in business with me for the duration; has a pace maker for a congenital heart condition; does yoga, tennis, and treadmill; and will be with me in business and as my life partner until the time we cast our last line in the ocean of opportunity.

For us our most productive life truly has begun with our commitment to a life style of love and family. However, looking around at our peers, the future is not so bright; most people our age opted for early retirement, do little if any exercise, have bad food choices, accept being overweight, are out of work, and are unhappy. To us this is not the American dream. It is going to be a nightmare for our economy, our health care system, and our children who will have to suffer with us in our old age and a society that thinks living unhappily past sixty-five is all we can expect. I have nothing but hope for our situation and nothing but fear for the majority of aging Americans that are going to expect to be housed, fed, diaper changed, and pushed around in a wheelchair.

If this sounds self-serving, it is. Our political system, economics, and work life are predicated on each of us pursuing happiness in a free and democratic society so we can retire early with no financial obligations, and not being institutionalized because we failed to prepare for aging. But our politicians, big government, and employers do not act in the best interests of the big picture. Spend now, worry later; avoid taxes, borrow more; and use credit to fund the high life now, apply for Medicaid later. Tax the folks and milk the goats for income, not outcome.

Strive to balance of work, relaxation and sleep for your 168 hours per week. 40 hours of work, 40 hours of relaxation, 48 hours of sleep per week, 40 hours for study and family. When you look at it this way we have plenty of time for balance if we use it properly.

The following book proposes a different approach for Aging in America with proposed structural changes and broader thinking on processes. Without those that are aging rethinking their life style and habits we are relegated to imposed theories by Government. This is the worst possible resolution. With massive numbers of citizens being warehoused and end of life care being rationed out it is moving us to a society of Soylent Green machines as depicted in the 1973 futuristic movie directed by Richard Fleischer and starring Charlton Heston and, in his final film, Edward G. Robinson, where they recycled elderly and disabled people into a green substance for feeding 40 million people in New York City.

PART I

Red Zone Habits In Pursuit of the Self-Health End Zone

CHAPTER ONE

What exactly is the Red Zone?

A <u>Red Zone</u> is a reference to decimated areas through war or military conflict smack dab in the middle of a violent and dangerous neighborhood, while it is a terrible area, people living there wouldn't change it or move if they could.

In football parlance The Red Zone is the space inside the twenty yard line . . . within reach of the Goal and a touchdown but with a challenge due to the shortened field of play and the pressure to succeed looming over the team. The Self-Health in football would be to score a touchdown versus a field goal. Why wouldn't you always get into the Self-Health Zone by being that close? Is it physical, mental or overcoming doubt? The winners of the game are the teams that move from the Red Zone past the goal line most consistently. And in my opinion it is more mental than physical by having the confidence to take chances and out fox the opponent.

In everyday life we all end up in the Red Zone by living on the edge of being healthy or being unhealthy due to how we view our lives. Thinking drives everything in the Red Zone. You are going to be healthy or unhealthy strictly on how you think about getting fit and staying fit. This is not intended to be a threat but a reality. Typical Red Zone thinking that results in a fumble and no shot at the Self-Health, is "I don't have time to exercise", "I

3

hate exercise", "I'm going to start", I don't have the money for a gym memberships, "I after I stop smoking", "I am down to two cigarettes per day and hope to quit entirely next week", "I hate fruits and vegetables", "I exercise and don't get any results", "I love to drink beer and eat potato chips only on Sunday watching sports on the couch with my dog", "I am too depressed to exercise", "I used to exercise then I got over weight and don't have the energy to even walk", etc. Only a small percentage of teams are successful in managing the Red Zone but they are the winners 100% of the time.

Don't take this wrong but these excuses are real and damaging to moving out of the Red Zone into the Self-Health of being fit, well, happier, more positive, more productive, a better spouse, friend or employee. It all starts with your thinking . . . because you are what you think you are. If you think fat you will be fat . . . if you think thin you will eventually be thin . . . if you are fat you will die younger than you should and if you are thin you have a chance to be disease free and have a happier, healthier prosperous life . . . that's the Self-Health . . . not my facts but the facts of eons of experts on how the mind works and how the body avoids work.

The mind is your most valuable asset and your body the neglected liability until we balance Red Zone work with Self-Health results.

Quotable Quotes:

> "Obesity is a curable disease of the mind." (Train the mind's conscious feelings about good subconscious habits that control the body's natural weight and biorhythm).

> "We used to think, there's nothing you can do about aging. You just age". (Now there's a feeling that it might be possible to slow it down).

"Aging isn't a curable disease it's a process. You need to know about the biological clock, oxidation and genes to manage the process." (Now it is diet for living longer, exercise for living better, and balance for living well).

"Food is the fuel for a longer lasting engine." (Now fruits, vegetables, red wine, dark chocolate, vitamin E, D and A, protein replacement, restraint for sugar, salt, white based products, portion control, micronutrient and calorie counting are the science of living longer).

"Exercise is the cure for a smoother running engine." (Cardio stimulation, strength training, resistance exercises, aggressive walking, deep breathing, yoga, stretching, meditation are fuel for the stronger engine are the science of living better).

"A study was conducted at a nursing home in Orange City, Florida. Nineteen men and women with an average age of 89, most of whom used wheelchairs to get around in, did just ten minutes of strength training per week. After 14 weeks almost everybody was out of their wheelchairs. One woman moved back into independent living." The results were published in Mature Fitness. If this is true for the elderly for 10 minutes per week what would it take to get 20% to 30% improvement for all ages?

MY AMERICA

My America is the feeling of freedom. It's the feeling good when you get up in the morning and can decide what you're going to do that day, who you're going to see and what you're going to say.

It's the feeling that you can make a difference. It's the feeling you can produce your product, you can sell

5

your produce and you can benefit from your hard work, unhindered. It's the feeling when you help your children with their homework, so they will be able to use their knowledge for growth, for maturity, for the good of the country. It's the feeling when you send them off to school, knowing they will receive a concerned teacher's attention, sensitivity and guidance. And knowing as they grow up, they will thrive on their freedom to communicate, to express themselves, to direct their own destiny.

It's the feeling when they graduate from grade school, junior high and high school that they are taking the steps towards a better life. And when you give their hand away in matrimony, that happiness shall be theirs. For together as husband and wife, they can create the same and even more opportunities for their off-spring.

It's that feeling when, you can unchain your dog and watch her run free for at least a little while, to watch the experience on her face, when she's released from the shackles; and the sadness that reappears when she must be chained.

My America is the freedom of choice to buy the bread I want to buy, to acquire the goods I can afford to acquire, to invest the capital I have saved, in ventures I want to take for the good of my family and my country.

My America is being able to communicate in writing, speaking and in whatever form, language takes, my opinions, my thoughts, my prayers, my visions and my dreams to those who want to listen, and to those enemies of the American way who in themselves have not discovered America.

My America is the blooming rose which has the freedom to grow towards, a clear sky and a warm sun; being able to complete its cycle from bloom to plumage to autumn to a dormant grave, only to rise again.

My America is the personal commitment to grab opportunities which will better the country and to set an example for those who follow; what you give, must be proportionate to what you take, or the erosion shall remove the sky, the sun, the earth from our grasp.

For in our America and the world resources are limited; the energy, though absolute, is redistributed by our wills. The more astute, the more free we are to create, the better the use of the resources. And left in God's hands, through our America, we create good will, good products, good people and peace of mind.

My America, oh yes my America, the vision of the poet, the words of the orator and minds of the leaders be kind, be patient, be wise, but above all be humble to the reasons and the heritage of our freedom. Lead us not into temptation, but deliver us from evil ventures and purposes, for thine America is the Kingdom, the power and the glory, forever. Amen.

It is also you and I wondering what will happen if we die early and leave no legacy. Why not leave a legacy of being fit as a habit not an illusion. The Self-Health mindset is a legacy of feeling good that succeeds over feeling guilty. Why not leave your offspring rising not falling far from the tree.

It is you and I not making changes in our attitude and life styles though we know we should. The Self-Health mindset is knowledge of self and the subconscious mind control over every action and every reaction. Ideas leading to happiness result from a healthy body and mind.

It is you and I not wanting to contemplate our demise so we avoid the commitment by allowing our bad habits to be our excuse and conductor. The Self-Health mindset is to focus on living every moment rather than dreading each day. Because it is thought that creates not circumstances. Thinking bad of anyone is going to make you think bad about your relationship with everyone.

We find in our scary waning years that the formation of life's expectancies are usually environmental, impulsive and reactionary. That is the Red Zone persona. All of us have it and need to shuck it. However, most of us will not because it takes a significant change in habits and life style.

OBAMA CARE RED ZONE THINKING

ACO's (Accountable Care Organizations), CCP's (Continuing Care Providers), QIO's (Quality Improvement Organizations), bundled payment, managed populations, enforcement penalties, taxes, taxes, more taxes are the proposed components of Obama Care. This concept of managed cost rather than managed quality is another brain child of the academics. Meaning that the resources will be Government's contribution to cover the cost not benefits based. The Government purchasers will pay a capitation rate (so much for a population grouping) and the continuum of care will have to collectively share in the limited monies.

> In theory the physician and hospital, if in control of the capitation payments from the Government, could conceivably make money by not admitting patients but merely referring them to others in the so called "continuum of care" . . . that unlucky business now has sicker patients with limited funding and extreme enforcement rules because they are dependent on the upper feeder who controls the bottom feeder.

Though quality is touted as being the driving force in funding it is cost not care that will drive the allocation of monies. It will still be treatment income not wellness outcomes that is foundation of the so called evidence based system. Pay for performance will then be based on providers' income not effective patient restorative outcomes. Inductive processes will delegate the responsibilities with transparency being an after the money is spent ineffective control mechanism. Business Enterprise will be pushed further to the background even though computer technologies are based on standardized business practices and deductive processes.

PATIENT PROTECTION AND AFFORDABLE CARE ACT (i.e., Obama Care)

Affordable—Not . . . Protecting the elderly and disabled—Not

Projected Cost = $465 Billion for State Exchanges
$434 Billion Medicaid Increases
$176 Billion Demonstration Projects and Enforcement
$1.075 Trillion Annul Coat

Projected Funding = $414 Billion Medicare Cuts
$349 Billion Provider Taxes
$210 Billion Medicare Withholding Taxes and Surtaxes
$107 Billion Pharmacy, Hospital Taxes
$ 68 Billion Fines and Penalties
$150 Billion Cadillac Insurance Taxes
$ 13 Billion Downsizing Medical Savings Accounts
$ 20 Billion Taxes on Devices
$ 15 Billion Reductions in Tax Deduction for Medical Expenses
$ 3 Billion Taxes on Tanning Salons

Jerry Rhoads

$1.218 Trillion Annual Taxes and Reductions
in Benefits

Projected, in theory is for the next decade but those types of forecasts are rarely in the ballpark when realty sets in . . . i.e. Medicare in its inception was to be costing in the millions not billions as is true of Part D medication coverage that will exceed $700 billion per year as the Boomers come on stream.

WHY OBAMA CARE WILL FAIL

First and foremost the Administration did lie about the cost and the loss of current insurance . . . leading to further lies about ease of registration and portability of coverage. Secondly, definitions of coverage will be left to bureaucrats since the Government is only funding a contribution to the cost not providing a benefit. Thirdly, managed care was tried in the late 1980's and early 1990's and it failed miserably because the principles were to squeeze cost of care not improve care processes to be more cost effective and efficient.

Why? Enterprise has been squeezed out of the equation. It is again a bureaucratic solution to personal health decisions that are controlled by the individual not Blue Zones, employers or the IRS. Why? Government is not accountable for performance standards and cannot execute evidence based systems. Ben Stein in his article "Don't Fear Corporations" states . . . Corporations in our era do not start wars, or crucify people, or send women and children to death camps. No, only governments that people, who hate corporations, love (usually because they are envious of the guts it takes to run a business and crave the security that government seems falsely to offer) commit atrocities. Corporations give us most of the good things we enjoy day by day in the way of material goods and services and do it in a usually effective, law abiding way. The governments and political that go after them are the ones to fear.

10

Why Singapore's health care system beats Obama Care

Singapore's health care system is just the opposite to Obama Care. It is built on a platform of individual responsibility for health preservation, prevention and wellness. Individuals pay for their own health preservation and care. It is an Enterprise model similar to my SHIFT system. It embraces savings accounts, spending decisions by the individual and a payment system managed by the Government. There are safety nets for the elderly and free health care for the poor who are responsible for their own health and wellness profile.

What are the metrics that prove Singapore's health care system is working better than any other approach in the world.

Singapore's life expectancy is superior:

Nation	Life Expectancy
Singapore	82
Australia	81.5
Canada	81.2
Japan	81
France	80.5
Sweden	80.5
Switzerland	80.5
Germany	79.5
United Kingdom	78.5
USA	78

Singapore's costs as a percent of GNP is superior to America.

Health Expenditures	
Nation	% of GDP
USA	16%
Singapore	3.25%
Canada	9%
Japan	8%
Germany	10%
United Kingdom	8%

Government share of the spending is reduced to a manageable level and accomplishing the objective of having a public option and a single payer system using the savings accounts administered by the Government but the spending decisions left with the individuals.

The savings accounts are the backbone for this Enterprise Model of health care because it introduces supply and demand and competition to the equation. This does not occur in America where someone else is responsible for making the buying and paying decisions. Where an insurance company or the Government pays the bill the individual does not internalize the necessity to stay fit and practice wellness habits.

My Proposed SHIFT SYSTEM (Self-Health Insurance Funding Trust) embodies the Enterprise Model and will produce the same results that are being demonstrated in Singapore.

AMERICA'S AGING AND HEALTH: IS IT A SCIENCE OR AN ART FORM?

Studies on the aging process and the poor health care picture are predicting a paradigm shift away from treatment to prevention and health preservation. Some studies show an increase in longevity and others that predict obesity and disease will cause the life expectancy to start a sharp decline. There is a diabolical struggle between science and socialized health care creating a Red Zone of need In Pursuit of proposed Self-Health Health and fitness solutions that require that an entire country change its personal living behaviors and habits. Predominately such dynamic movements in mores and habits takes decades . . . do we have that kind of time with the Boomers Coming at us at 7,000 per day?

Politically, who is on the right and the left on this problem? Is Obama Care a solution or an added burden? In the center what I see are the telltale signs of Americans not taking responsibility for their health and their ongoing aging costs. What is their responsibility and what are the tangible and intangible costs of aging?

Responsibilities and current status:

1) Americans need a healthier life style

   a. Fitness: 66% of Americans do not exercise even 10 minutes per week
   b. Nutrition: 45% of Americans do not read the labels on the containers
   c. Emotional Instability: 25% of Americans use some form of mind altering chemicals
   d. Stressors: 90% of Americans do not use exercise, relaxation, and meditation in their day
   e. Sleep deprivation: Average sleep is 6 hours

2) Americans need a healthier financial picture

   a. Financial under funding for the aging costs: Most Americans have pension benefits but no long term care insurance.
   b. No financial plan for nursing home care

Problems (Americans in general do not have healthy life styles):

Obesity (disease of the mind) and Chronic diseases (bad habits) head the list:

- Inactivity and lack of concern for personal health responsibilities
- Poor diet choices and no plan for improving their diet
- Prescription drug side-affects without knowing what they are
- Stressful relationships resulting in divorce and unhappiness
- Chronological age is less then biological age and widening
- Externalize responsibility for wellness and do not internalize the consequences
- Government programs ration out the money to the providers for treating the symptoms
- Acquired infections and chemical use destroy the immune system
- Smoking destroys all body systems over time

#1 Problem: Most Americans ride everywhere. They are generally not fit. Little if no walking is required in our society. Studies show that 15 to 20 minutes per day of brisk walking will prevent many maladies and improve the longevity by 20%. Yet no one walks anywhere unless they have to.

#2 Problem: Most Americans eat whatever is put in front of them without regard to nutritional content or side-effects on their health. Obesity is a growing health problem due to the American life style. It is rippling to our next generation.

#3 Problem: Most Americans do not get enough sleep and use medication for rest and relaxation.

#4 Problem: Most Americans have 40 to 50 hour per week jobs and other time demanding activities resulting in stressful 14 to 16 hour days.

#5 Problem: 50% of Americans are getting divorced.

#6 Problem: Most Americans do not prepare for the aging process. Getting old is for someone else and I will worry about it if it happens to me some day. Studies show there are more young people with diabetes, heart conditions, plugged arteries, shortness of breath, osteoporosis, joint diseases, emotional instabilities, social maladies, etc. As these people exacerbate the diseases with weight problems the hospital and nursing home are not far away.

#7 Problem: Most Americans have someone else paying for their insurance and are not responsible for funding the services to treat their poor life styles. This builds in over utilization of a cost based system.

#8 Problem: The Government is administering 80% of the health care benefits with only 60% of the resources needed to pay for an aging and unhealthy population. This is catching up with the State Medicaid programs that now want to ration health care. Medicare is using enforcement and fear to keep their costs down.

#9 Problem: Acquired infections and chemical use. We continue to put foreign substances in our bodies and wonder why we have respiratory conditions, sinus infections, headaches, bowel impaction, bladder leaking, aberrant blood sugars, flu like symptoms, stomach and intestinal complications, cancer, diabetes, heart conditions, collapsed lungs, prostate infections, etc.

#10 Problem: smoking is killing 5 million people per year and we ignore the fact that the smokers die, on average, 20 years sooner than nonsmokers . . . it costs us all $5 billion per year in health care services for the smokers who also generate the above 8 problems with their externalized self-inflicted problem.

Solutions (Life styles come more easily with a system to follow) Aging needs to be a treated as a Science rather than an Art form:

- There needs to be a personal commitment to health as a life style.
- There needs to be professional help to set up programs for fitness, nutrition, relaxation activities, vacation, sleep patterns, family counseling for troubles in the marriage, etc.
- There needs to be standardized benefits structured for the personal health care needs
- There needs to be economic incentives for getting to the above 3 moral incentives to preserve health and pursue outcomes for unhealthy Americans.

    - Tax incentives for investing in a healthy life style
    - Membership at a fitness center
    - Attention to diet using nutritional counseling
    - Acquit ion and use of fitness equipment
    - Attention to physical health using a personal trainer
    - Attention to relationships using a marriage counseling
    - Use of sleep studies and therapeutic devices for rest and relaxation
    - Managed weight loss and stop smoking programs using health coaches
    - Use of screening for respiratory, urinary, bone, arterial, mental and emotional problems

- There needs to be less governmental intervention and more private sector controls

- o Pretax withholding of long term care insurance premiums for working Americans
- o Nonworking and under insured Americans funded thru traditional Medicaid programs
- o Elderly Americans that have a need for hospitalization and crisis intervention would be funded thru the traditional Medicare Programs
- o Providers of health preservation services would be paid on an outcome basis using fitness plan templates and proof of interventions and goals reached.
- o Providers of health care services would also be paid on an outcome basis using care plan templates and proof of interventions and goals reached for

  - Physical problems
  - Motor problems
  - Emotional Problems
  - Social Problems

- Life expectancy planning and health preservation services then become the mode of managing costs and benefits. They are the new enterprises. Capital investment and return from earnings should be based on outcomes not everyone's incomes. Right now the life expectancy is a turkey shoot and the costs are fraught with waste and corruption.

My Story in the Red Zone:

Born in a small town in Indianola Iowa I felt small, thought big and lived in between . . . liking sports because of feeling good about accomplishment and equal to or better than the others playing. School was necessary and fairly easy. My memories of Hawthorn Grade School are about the recesses and the girls . . . very little about studies or future.

Jerry Rhoads

Brought up in a lower middle class neighborhood by depression era parents did not inspire the bright lights of Des Moines and the other cities were not even on my mind map.

Junior High School was a big step up because I began to learn stimulating subjects . . . geography opened up the whole world . . . algebra opened up my mind to solving problems . . . science opened up my life to the underlying meaning of living . . . English allowed me to start writing . . . government stimulated my first poem about the Russian premier Georgi Boletnikov and his takeover of the Communist Politburo . . . track made me realize that running sprints was not my strength but distance was . . . girls on the other hand were being forced on me by my friends because of my height (5'1" in eight grade) and shyness . . . since I was in love with my baseball glove (a Rawlings infielder model) and looked like Mr. Peepers with by horned rim glasses girls did not see me like I saw them . . . then Sharon White came into focus in front of the Junior High early in 1954 . . . blond, cute, very attractive figure in my eyes and distant. Not knowing about the Laws of Attraction I only thought of the "what if's" . . . what if she doesn't like me . . . what if she laughs when I say hello . . . what if her friend Rosie tells her about my being a shrimp . . . will my best friend Sam take her away from me before I have a chance to grow taller.

Fast forward to High School and the departure of Sharon White to Brooklyn, Iowa where her father got a new job . . . no one to dream about . . . the girls my friends pushed me towards were too tall or too skinny or too ugly or too smart or too "stuck up".

My red zone thinking was being triggered by a lower middle class family environment of life being circumstantial . . . if you are poor to mildly poor without hope of being on the north side of a small town or belonging to the country club or a member of the Methodist church you were on the outside looking in and wondering if the big city would be better. Sports opened the door to me having hope of being exceptional and attaining a bigger life and a better future. My problem was being too small according to the basketball coach, but my smallness was embraced by the football coach because of my courage to challenge the bigger guys and a baseball coach that respected my abilities at shortstop (best hands I have ever seen), so hope blossomed.

Unfortunately, my father who was pushing me to excel at baseball due to his interest in the sport, resulted in my finding out early that I was not good enough to go very far . . . so I played out my career in high school and never aspired for more, as I had in my younger days. The same was true in basketball . . . as the sixth man I displayed talent but did not meet the coaches view of a point guard that could out score his favored big guys. Football jettisoned me after my sophomore year because my parents could not afford the required athletic insurance of $3 and I dropped out . . . becoming the team manager just to stay close to a sport I loved.

Graduation came in 1957 with me wondering what to do to get out of Indianola and feel good about my life. For some reason Sharon and I had the same aspirations but did not know it until we were brought together on Halloween night in 1956 when Nancy suggested that the three of us go to the haunted house towards Pleasantville . . . as we approached the house Sharon grabbed hold of me and the rest is history . . . we starting dating and have been together (except for 9 months when she went to cosmetology school in Dubuque) ever since (54 years of marriage, 4 great children, 12 Grandchildren, one great/great grandson and going for 80 years together).

Next came college with me feeling inadequate and not so smart . . . I graduated in the top 1/3 of the class but nothing spectacular. The first semester passed with me getting ordinary grades (2.7) with little hope of being the dreams I had in sports. The second semester I took the required course that I had a C in the first semester . . . psychology. The professor was considered impossible for good grades and a C was the best he gave . . . but all of a sudden I found a desire and interest in Plato, Aristotle and their use of logic.

Lo and behold I got A's on the exams and an A for the semester . . . the only one and considered to be a miracle. Somehow this triggered my next three years in college to excel at my studies . . . only I could control that and it worked. I ended with a B+ average for the four years and 3.75 for my last two years. I was selected for special recognition and studies in the humanities and received the Wall Street Journal award for the outstanding business graduate in 1961 . . . headed to the big city of Chicago as a recruit with Arthur Andersen & Co . . . the best CPA firm in the world.

But fear still prevailed because I still lived my dreams in reverse . . . wanting to excel at sports as the fulfillment of my desire to be the best at something . . . hating my inadequacies when it came to my job and knowing that there was something wrong with me when it came to auditing and bean counting. I felt that it was my lack of talent when in affect it was not logical to me to just check out and correct other people's mistakes . . . then I got a call from the Personnel Department of AA&Co. and was transferred to the Small Business Division of the Chicago Office.

Just as Sharon White and Freshman Psychology changed my life, so did this not so subtle change in my career path . . . I was now able to use some of my emerging creativity to do tax planning for my clients and advise them on the economics of business not just fixing the books. Computers came on the scene and I learned how to use the applications and automate those messy books so they were more accurate. We developed inventory systems, marketing plans, stock capitalization plans, corporate organization charts, team building, documentation systems and behavior psychology for hiring and managing employees. This was s great education in entrepreneurship. I credit this as the first move into the Self-Health for me and my family.

Health care came into my life as a career focus when I was assigned to the Blue Cross of America account to audit hospitals in1962 and help roll out Medicare in 1967 and Medicaid in 1968 . . . now 45 years later these skills that I developed at AA&Co. deliver me every day to the market place with hope for bringing Self-Health habits to an aging society. In 1968 I passed the CPA exam and left Arthur Andersen and Chicago in 1969 for greener pastures with a small CPA firm. Then after four years of consulting for Catholic Hospital chains I moved on to another CPA firm that wanted me as the Partner in Charge of their health care practice.

Over the years in the Red Zone of health care I worked for CPA firms in Springfield and Peoria, Illinois, that were in it for the money, started my own CPA firm in 1977, expanded that business into consulting, software development and proposed public offering for capital to take my ideas to a higher level. The economy took a downturn during the Carter years when interest rates for my SBA loan and bank line of credit went to 23% and I had to sell off the accounting firm and consulting practice to save the software in a Chapter 11 bankruptcy filing.

So we relocated back to Chicago and the enterprise was restarted as an accounting firm specializing in nursing homes. During my four years in Springfield, Illinois, the capitol of Illinois I gained notoriety as an expert in Medicare and Medicaid regulations for nursing homes . . . was the lead consultant for the trade associations and expert witness for legislation protecting the owners' interest. When we returned to Chicago many of my contacts in the politics of nursing homes engaged me as a consultant to help them lobby and file their cost reports. My business again flourished but my dreams did not.

The Self-Health software systems we developed during my years in Morton, Illinois (a suburb of Peoria) and financed with the SBA and bank lines was saved by my Chapter 11 filing became my albatross . . . being programmed in an outdated language and utilizing mini computers rather than PC's destined us to miss the mark even though the design was and still is revolutionary. Then my son Kip got involved in the business and slowly brought us into the PC world with new software. For the next 20 years we traveled around the country installing different versions of the system in 141 different nursing homes in 22 different states . . . enabling the operators to bring Medicare into their business as a way to restore patients back to their homes.

But in our estimation this effort did not bring the nursing homes into the Self-Health but took them to the Green Zone of prosperity . . . money flowed, reputations glowed, but quality patient care did not. The system that I dreamed of was not performing the way it was designed . . . get 'em in, get 'em better and get 'em back home . . . rather it created a way for the businesses (usually run by real estate moguls) to fill the beds and make more profit for the owners . . . who then would sell the business to a larger chain that would make even more money. Even though the Federal Government used punitive methods to keep the reimbursement down our system and documentation (directed by the Federal Courts) forced them to pay for the care. Neither, in my opinion, were contributing to the restoring of health for the elderly and disabled.

So we decided to get out of that business and into operating nursing homes utilizing our systems, knowledge and dream of providing aging America a quality of life not just a room, diaper, TV and bad food. We are now setting up the Self-Health mentally in long term care by using outcome driven systems and procedures to reduce over medication, improve function and create hope for a return to the community . . . in 57% of the cases we have successfully discharged admissions back home. The 43% who must stay have a quality of life that revolves around their Activities of Daily Living being managed for an ACTIVE continuum of life. We are extending lives not just ending them in a depressing nursing home . . . I like to say we are managing life not death.

However, our pursuit has been fraught with the bureaucracy refusing to change to a positive and collaborative approach to compliance and the result is retaliation that is on the verge of putting us out of business because they can. There will be more on this later. See Appendix II for the bloody realities of Big Government's sustaining the RED ZONE.

IT's HELL TO BE OLD (AUTHOR UNKNOWN)

"I can't chew raw carrots, celery or cabbage and sometimes the meat is burned and dried. I don't like it when the food is all jumbled together; it makes me sick to look at it. Often, they spill the coffee and milk so I only have a couple of mouthfuls left to drink. Have you ever tried to eat dry pancakes for supper? If only I could explain why I can't eat".

I used to have a whole house of my own, but now my world has shrunk to this little area of my bed and chair. Most nurses are respectful of my area, treating the few things I have left with care, but others are like some bold children who visited in my home once and pawed through my drawers and broke my antique vase. Some of the people here remind me of the neighborhood bullies who thought the world was theirs for the taking and knocked down anyone in their way.

Another thing that is devastating is to have my room changed. Time and time again I see a friend hauled off to a new eight by six area in a strange room. Sometimes it happens to me: suddenly, without warning, a caravan of nurses and aides will appear and begin taking clothes from my closet in preparation for the move. All of us dread this happening.

I need to know when I get out of my bed in the morning, that I can get back into that same bed at night. Some days I'm so afraid I won't be able to, that I resist getting up. Sometimes I refuse to go for a walk in the hall because it may be a ruse to move me into another room. If I have to move again, I think it will break my heart.

I've had a hard life—never much money, many clothes, or possessions. I'm not extravagant. I have known depression days and times of hunger and I have mended the patches on my clothes. Is it any wonder that I like to have a small piece of bread or cracker in my purse just in case there is no food tomorrow, or in case I get hungry tonight? There's no pantry or icebox I can go to. Sometimes an aide brings a cup of juice or milk, but nothing to eat. "It makes crumbs", she says, or, "Well, you should have eaten your supper. Then you wouldn't be hungry"

Sometimes I look deep into the eyes of a nurse and ask, "How would you like to be me?" I can remember back to my youth when I never gave a thought to growing old and I think these youngsters who are nurses are doing today what I did then: they are hiding—from thoughts of old age. They don't really want to look at me—to know me—because in me, they would see themselves as they will someday and they don't want to do that. Some—day you'll be just like me, I want to say to them when I'm feeling bitter. "Will you remember then another little old lady a long time ago who said, "How would you like to be me?"

"Never Too Old to Live" (a Self-Health book)

- Jerry Rhoads' latest book prescribes making the changes that the Self-Health principles propose.
- His 10 chapters give doable regimens for attaining the 10 Self-Health commandments.
- His tools assist in downsizing your waist size and up scaling your activity to improve your self-worth and BMI.
- His mental exercising as a Self-Health action is taking your subconscious to task and changing the way you are thinking about yourselves and your life style outcomes.

- His seminars on Self-Health are taking Americans to Self-Health status. The goal is to allow us all to break 100.

My departure from the Red Zone consists of 10 personal self-health Commandments using a stop and start sign for approach to changing habits:

ONE   Stop negative thinking, start feeling good
TWO   Stop eating whatever you desire, start eating for joy
THREE Stop being a couch potato, start being an action hero
FOUR   Stop hating your job, sports team, financial situation, start loving your life
FIVE   Stop finding fault with others, start finding more friends
SIX   Stop being angry with yourself, start feeling good, thinking well and being healthy
SEVEN Stop destructive habits that age you, start learning to control the subconscious impulses that control us
EIGHT Stop hunting for the better marriage, start renewing your feeling and power of love
NINE   Stop hunting for a better job, start working for others' dreams
TEN   Stop cynical complaining (about politics, religion, sex, taxes, money and social obstacles to your success), start being a part of the solutions

PLAN YOUR EPITAPH: You are Never too Old to Live, Always to Young to Die by not living a better way . . . Never Say Die . . . Always Think Young and the Years will take care of themselves For more on this departure from the Red Zone read my Book "Never Too Old to Live" . . . Xlibris 2012

What does the future hold? With 77 million baby boomers reaching retirement age and finding that retirement is not feasible and need to reverse bad living habits . . . we are focusing our services on wellness . . . and are campaigning that hospitals, physicians, therapists and nurses focus on functional outcomes (the Self-Health movement) not prescription drugs that mask improvement and tests, treatments and methods (the Red Zone tsunami) that have side-affects that compound the existing diagnosed problems.

Self-Health Exercises . . . the Self-Health of life is not restricted to waking hours or how you spend your work hours . . . it is how you spend your nonworking hours. There are usually 14 per day, 84 per week, 350 per month, 4,200 per year and approximately 327,600 in your life time. 6 to 8 hours per day is for sleeping or 199,200 hours in a lifetime. This leaves 128,310 hours of free time for whatever you decide to do with your life. This is 14 hours of wellness, fitness, lowering stress opportunities . . . do we usually use them that way . . . none of us do so religiously. Why not? Each person has to answer that but even sleep can be more productive if we are stress free. Does eating the right foods do it? Does a good love life do it? Does a satisfying job do it? Does making a fortune do it? Does being a celebrity do it? I think we can agree that the answer is no way.

Try this for a change: commit to going from Red Zone thinking to Self-Health living . . . Chapter Two has the answer to a life style generated by fasting the Red Zone habits into Self-Health living.

Profile of a Red Zoner

- Overweight (from 200 pounds to 1,000 +)
- In mid-forties to fifties a smoker and heavy drinker with a life expectancy if lucky of 70 to 75 with last years in a nursing home
- Avoids doctors but is sick at least one day per week
- Is a chronic complainer and is on the second or third marriage
- Is cynical about sports, politics and chick movies (the male Red Zoner)

- Is dependent on facials, botox, tummy tucks, diets and fantasies (the female Red Zoner)
- Uses emergency care quite often due to indigestion, palpitations, trouble breathing, out of whack blood sugars

DOWNSIZER

With the average weight of Americans, at all ages in the Red Zone, escalating at a troublesome rate we must formulate solutions that move individuals to their ideal BMI. My Downsizer is a failsafe tool to direct the reduction of weight by increasing physical activity for mental fitness.

Weights by category:
More than two-thirds (68.8 percent) of adults are considered to be overweight or obese.
More than one-third (35.7 percent) of adults are considered to be obese.
More than 1 in 20 (6.3 percent) have extreme obesity.
Almost 3 in 4 men (74 percent) are considered to be overweight or obese.
The prevalence of obesity is similar for both men and women (about 36 percent).
About 8 percent of women are considered to have extreme obesity.

Obesity is predicted to be the highest cause of premature death, chronic disease and over utilization of health care services. Obesity is considered to be a disease of the mind rather than the body. To help those that decide to become what they want to be I have developed the downsizer formula tied to exercise processes that each individual can choose and plan their weight reduction and attainment of their desired BMI. Just click on the link www.americaintheredzone.com to access the downsizer tool.

CHAPTER TWO

What exactly is a Self-Health End Zone Diet?

From the best-selling book The Blue Zones author and explorer Dan Buettner chronicles the "Lessons for Living Longer from the People Who've Lived the Longest with the right lifestyle, experts say, chances are that you may live up to a decade longer. What's the prescription for success? National Geographic Explorer Dan Buettner has traveled the globe to uncover the best strategies for longevity found in the Blue Zones: places in the world where higher percentages of people enjoy remarkably long, full lives. In this dynamic book he discloses the recipe, blending this unique lifestyle formula with the latest scientific findings to inspire easy, lasting change that may add years to your life."

The book's research in the Blue Zones found nine common characteristics of all the world's longest-lived people.

1. Move naturally . . . walking instead of riding, exercise the body and brain
2. Have a Purpose . . . work for something or someone
3. Slow down . . . smell the roses
4. Eat what you like, stop when you're full . . . avoid overeating

5. Eat plant life for micro nutrients rather than meats . . . weight is a function of intake and output
6. Moderate consumption of Wine . . . preferably red
7. Socialize . . . belong to something
8. Put Loved Ones first . . . love is rewarding
9. Pick your friends carefully . . . the social networks matter

"To make it to age 100, you have to have won the genetic lottery. But most of us have the capacity to make it well into our early 90's and largely without chronic disease. As the Adventists demonstrate, the average person's life expectancy could increase by 10-12 years by adopting a Blue Zone lifestyle."

It is your life style in waiting for improved . . . .

— Thinking
— Acting
— Eating
— Loving
— Giving
— Believing
— Working
— Health
— Wealth
— Prosperity

It takes the activities of others in their worlds who have attained Self-Health status and gives the principles to you for your use in moving through the Red Zone. But first you have to change your thinking about longevity and changing your sub conscious unhealthy habits. You have to internalize the impact of good health not externalize it as not your responsibility as we have been brain washed to believe . . . it is a privilege not a right to be kept healthy.

Red Zone thinking habits infect us all from childhood due to our parents being stuck with it themselves. When do you remember them saying let's be nice for a day and give in to everyone we meet? Rather we hear:

- What happened to your allowance?
- Shut the door, were you born in a barn?
- Go ask your Mother.
- Don't talk like that to your Mother.
- Okay, but don't tell your Mother I let you.
- You're grounded.
- That's my chair you are sitting in.
- As long as you're living in this house, you live by my rules.
- You don't know how good you have it.
- This is going to hurt me more than it hurts you.
- Who left my tools out?
- Who opened two bottles of milk.
- Don't slam the door.
- If you don't cut that out I will ground you.
- I'll give you something to cry about.
- Turn that thing down.
- I'm not sleeping I am just resting my eyes.
- Turn on the lights do you want to ruin your eyes.
- I'm only going to say this one more time.
- I get no respect around here.
- Do as I say not as I do.
- Do you think I'm made of money?
- Who left the bicycle in the driveway?
- You don't know how good you have it.
- Don't slam the door one more time.
- Why didn't you go before we left?
- Because I said so.
- Don't talk back or I will keep the car keys.
- Eat your dinner . . . there are people starving in Africa.

Red Zone talk creates a Red Zone way of habitual thinking . . . I can't, I don't, I won't until we are only creating problems rather than solving them. Why is it better to talk about I can, I do, I will? Our minds work on our words and the words of others. For example:

> I can't hit a golf ball . . . I have never tried . . . I never will.
> I can hit a golf ball . . . I want to try . . . I will succeed.
>
> I don't believe in God . . . It doesn't make sense to me . . . It won't save me anyway.
> I do believe in the Super natural . . . It is important that I believe . . . This will help me be positive. Even though I am not able to prove God . . . it gives me hope.
>
> I won't give in to that person . . . she's disgusting and mean . . . I hate her.
> I will try to talk to her . . . she isn't too bad when she smiles . . . I probably can like her.

Self-Health habitual talking and thinking sets the ball rolling to communication, exchange of feelings and eventually understanding . . . what an asset when used to make friends, make love and create solutions to health problems.

Red Zone acting is the silent body language that communicates disgust rather than trust . . . disregard rather than regard for the other person's state of mind . . . rejection rather than reflection about their opinion, likes, dislikes and feelings. Self-Health acting embraces courtesy, caring about feelings, looking for chances to help, receiving compliments after giving them, finding good traits and looks in everyone.

Red Zone eating is without regard to the body's needs for the joy of fulfilling the five senses . . . unhealthy food is not just a bad habit it is a death warrant for a shortened life. It kills the sense of smell by creating a false sense of satisfaction . . . it kills the sight of food by just wanting the taste not the value of food . . . it destroys wanting to hear others tell you to change . . . it forces one to feel good about being wrong . . . and it limits taste to the tongue only. Self-Health eating contemplates the five senses before eating . . . the smell is not the reason for eating . . . it is the result of tasting something that is visually colorful and stimulates what others are saying about our habits.

Red Zone loving is the control of infatuation and misdirected sexual desires over giving of one's self-directed concern for the mate. The desire is to see rather than feel, the temptation to excite rather than to give, the disregard of giving rather than getting one's self-centered needs satisfied. Self-Health loving is the components of relationships that start slowly and mature from needing and wanting each other. In between, when there are setbacks, the Self-Health partnership takes precedent over ego and opinion. Marriage is just one facet of the Self-Health loving . . . but it is the most important . . . other facets are having children, having a successful sex life . . . having a long lasting respect for each other . . . in sickness and in health . . . until death do us part.

Red Zone giving comes with an agenda . . . if I give this will I get that . . . who else is going to give and will it be enough . . . I don't have it but I will fake it . . . sacrifice may be what I have to do . . . hold them accountable if I give it to them . . . Charities are for the rich . . . the rich should be the benefactors. Self-Health giving is without thought . . . it is a reflex . . . it is a desire to help . . . it is the difference between those that have respect and those that are worried about money . . . it is the satisfaction of making things better for everyone.

Red Zone believing holds out until there are signs of receiving . . . there is no vision nor since of mission or responsibility for others . . . therefore, it is not belief it is looking for relief of fear and distrust . . . it is easier to be doubtful than to work on making it happen . . . it is more realistic to be critical than it is to take the chance . . . it is not standing for something and falling for anything. Self-Health believing, on the other hand, is seeing before it happens . . . finding before looking . . . prospering while giving . . . staying on track when the road ends . . . filling up the hearts of others with hope and encouragement . . . growing crops while other blame the weather for their lack of results . . . leading others to the trough before it rains . . . talking of good times despite the black clouds of today . . . seeing the future and predicting all is well.

Red Zone working hates the thought of wasting time on problem solving . . . looks forward to time off . . . wants to retire early, afford it or not . . . view vacation as the best days of one's life . . . finds others success distasteful . . . criticizes those that want to advance . . . second guesses those that take risks . . . blames circumstance for failures . . . loves the week-ends and has blue Mondays each week. Self-Health working loves the thought of being productive . . . wants more and desires more than what is available today . . . isn't afraid of failure . . . looks to God as the Sheppard and the protector . . . fights off doubt through self-affirmation . . . confirms that the mind is the maker and the body is the enabler . . . values health, happiness and effort more than lotto, gambling at the casinos and death deifying tricks . . . works at everything in life.

Red Zone health gives into temptation . . . favors taste over value . . . takes chances with warning signals (sugar, salt, corn syrup, fat, carbs, alcohol, chocolate), of over indulgence in any facet of life . . . rationalizing body weight, BMI, waistline, chemical use, deviate behaviors, aberrant sexuality and negative thinking.

Self-Health health is a personal commitment to making a sacrifice for life style, wellness, exercise, and avoidance of the other side of everything thought good . . . those in the zone are not only focused on health they are positive about life's purpose and find joy in taking chances with natural remedies and health sciences that start with the cultivation of the mind's depth and control over the senses.

Red Zone Wealth is the destructive and misuse of the Enterprise System . . . cheating and breaking of the laws of mankind and the natural resources is a temporary reaping and raping of our natural desires to live happily, health and prosperously . . . those that steal from nature to profit have destroyed the earth's ability to sustain life . . . those that don't give back to the source of their wealth are destroying the fabric of Enterprise . . . whether it is our tax system, our laws, our political parties or our businesses the wealth produced should be the wealth replaced.

Self-Health does give back to the Enterprise by capitalizing the replacement of natural resources with investment in creative businesses, time saving technologies, better health remedies, restored respect for the elderly, more logical application of Government, more emphasis on fiscal policy directed by the majorities regardless of class and through better educational facilities for all.

Red Zone Prosperity is the rich getting richer and the poor getting poorer. No taxing system can correct this disparity. It must come from a reinvestment of the riches back into the very system that created the wealth. Taxing net worth will create the Self-Health economy. Letting the overhead of our Economy be dictated by a few politicians creates 40% of our resources being wasted on regulations and paperwork that destroys initiative and taxable revenues.

Self-Health prosperity comes from freedom to fail, recover and reinvest in ideas, new technologies, better remedies, fewer pills and prevention of chronic diseases . . . it is the overall health of our country that builds the future for Americans . . . since 35%

of population will be over 65 in 15 years the other 65% will be looking at the overhead and fixed costs to cut . . . that is called rationing of health care expenditure which destroys the fabric of taking care of those that cannot take care of themselves. On the other hand, taxing net worth will recapitalize the existing businesses and start the new businesses that create the new jobs . . . otherwise the use of taxes to protect the fixed overhead will destroy our ability to compete with the emerging economies that do not have 19.7 million government employers and a $1 trillion dollar nonproductive payroll . . . this situation is resulting in bankruptcy for the greatest economy in the world.

Will the Blue Zone cultural approach to America in the Red Zone? Is this a religious mass exodus based on change of the environment or an individual's commitment to their own longevity, happiness, prosperity and freedom to live well? I believe that cultural change is the least likely to succeed in the short run because our society is not focused on self-health but self-gratification. To theorize that we, as a mass of individual bad habits, can be converted to an Okinawa outcome does not focus on how we got to where we are in our ignorance of wellness. This again is bureaucratic thinking about a personal problem that needs the use of economic incentives not externalizing the problem and wanting the providers, employers, companies to produce results that the employees and citizens need to internalize.

The general attitude towards self-health is we don't have time to be healthy and how we eat, breathe, love, work, are responses to our subconscious that has been developed over the years by our relationships, environment, education, values, dreams and aspirations. Can this be changed by a Blue Zone campaign or a American in the Red Zone book . . . my opinion it will not.

However, we must start somewhere or perish as a nation chasing diets and quick fixes. My problem with the Blue Zone project is it inductive premise . . . if we change the surroundings and inputs the outputs should occur. This in fact could happen, but has yet to happen, over a period of 100 years as it has with the Blue Zones based on that compact set of mores without much mobility and change of venues. Looking back in history this approach has yet to work except for two occurrences . . . group movements are motivated by either fear or faith . . . the first was Hitler's movement using fear and the second, the most famous, was Jesus Christ's using sin as the reason for individual commitment and blind faith.

To recreate that defies the transient American modus operanti so the deductive approach can be more productive. American's must not fear their way into health nor use just statements of I will, I can and I am. We must think our way to health through stated goals for the following profile:

Profile of a Self-Health End Zone Winner

- Is a chronic positive thinker whose glass is half full and still in a stable marriage loving life and spouse and family and job and the Cubs
- Stabilize weight (from 100 pounds to 200—) eats right and thinks thin
- In mid-forties to fifties a nonsmoker and wine drinker with a life expectancy if lucky of 90 to 105 with no last years in a nursing home
- Sees few doctors and is never sick and takes vitamins rather than drugs
- Loves sports, and participates in politics and goes to the movies with his wife (the male Self-Health Zoner)
- Is not dependent on facials, botox, tummy tucks, diets and fantasies (the female Self-Health Zoner) the all-natural beautiful chick
- Uses no emergency care and quite often indulges in physical activities of people half their age such as exercise commitments for the mind and body

How do we know if American's in the Red Zone will actually pursue these outcomes? Since the moral incentives used by the Blue Zone Project are morally correct, only economic incentives get effective results . . . so if Obama Care wants the Blue Zones to spread across America through competition among communities and recognition without their commitment to pay for self-health habits will fail as other similar approaches have. Obama Care must define the outcomes that build a healthier America and then pay for those in the benefit package (not just a dollar commitment to contribute to the hope that Blue Zone type projects will inductively change American's bad habits in a mass exodus to a new healthier culture). It only took six decades of Government controls and laws to dumb down American's habits. On the other hand the "thinking diet" builds on positive thoughts to heal.

(See END NOTES (1)—(6) page 281 for the author's final take on the Blue Zone movement . . . according to their proponents the 8 Blue Zone cultures have never been successfully replicated in any community yet) . . . maybe ever.

CHAPTER THREE

Self-Health and Health Care Are Not a Right

- Being healthy is a privilege to be earned

  — We are Born to be free
  — We are Born to be a person
  — We are Born to be alive
  — But we Live and Die as we decide to be

- The privilege is earned by our habits, thoughts and actions every day . . . it is our own zone that determines our health, happiness and prosperity!

The Constitution of the United States:

We the People of the United States, in Order to form a more perfect Union, establish Justice, insure domestic Tranquility, provide for the common defense, promote the general Welfare, and secure the Blessings of Liberty to ourselves and our Posterity, do ordain and establish this Constitution for the United States of America.

No where in the constitution does it state that Government is responsible for the health of its citizens. It does state that the perfect

Union shall promote the general Welfare but not our physical, mental and financial health.

Defining the Health Care Problem

"You first need to define the problem before you can solve the Problem." Peter Drucker in "The Effective Executive" and Michael Gerber in the "E-myth Manager state that "no problem can be solved without an effective management system".

Hospitals beds	discharges	Patient days	Gross revenues	
4,027	757,232	32,799,020	152,308,338	$2,054,194,370

Hospitals over the last 25 years have built huge edifices of treatment . . . most used public funds and never paid one penny of taxes since they are not for profit . . . ha ha. Take 5,000 hospitals adding $150 million in physical buildings and equipment = $1,250,000,000,000 in expansion funded out of endowments, trust funds, public monies, contributions, insurance company pass through(s). This is generating $1,000,000,000,000 trillion in annual revenues that are not taxed at all. And they keep upping the prices and lowering the quality of life.

954,224 Physicians practicing in America make an average of $500,000 per year in fee for service = $450,000,000,000 billion and they want to make decisions on who to treat and when to avoid accountability and insist that their medicine is defensive due to lawsuits holding them accountable for their art form of health care (pursuit of treatment and medication first and outcome only if it fits their need for income). They would love Tort Reform rather than so called Health Care Reform. "Give us more money and we will give you quality health care."

2,909,357 **licensed registered nurses** 752,300 licensed practical nurses practicing in America make an average of $50,000 per year and are focused on treatment more than prevention since they take their orders from the physicians. Much of their time is spent passing prescription drugs and performing treatments to assist in the remedy of illnesses.

350 health insurance companies passing all their costs that are not controlled at all by accountability or performance, onto the unsuspecting employers and employees at the rate of $1,300,000,000,000 trillion per year that erodes our economy's ability to compete with foreign companies while they profit to the tune of $130,000,000,000 billion per year with no accountability to quality or performance . . . fortunately they gladly pay income taxes at a rate of 28% after loop holes and lobbyists.

33,000 pharmacies billing for 8 billion medications passed in nursing homes, 5 billion in hospitals and 2 billion in other health care providers at a rate of $25 per script = $375,000,000,000 billion charged to Medicare, Medicaid, insurance companies and private parties with no accountability nor measure of performance . . . just their earnings per share that erodes our economy when the medications are contra indicated and/or flushed down the toilet in nursing homes due to over medication and erroneous diagnosis due to 95% of the orders being made over the telephone without a doctor's evaluation of outcome or side-affects.

16,100 nursing homes with 86% occupancy are paid an average of $3,500,000 per year by Medicare and Medicaid for rent, poor food, a bed and a wheelchair that costs the government $750,000,000 to supply. That is a whopping $48,000,000,000 billion per year plus private insurance and self-pay insurers another $34,000,000,000 billion per year for poor quality of life and shortened end of life results.

1.7 million elderly are warehoused in the 16,100 nursing homes and are re-hospitalized on an average of 4 times per year or 5,800,000 admissions to hospitals per year . . . each hospitalization costs Medicare, private insurance, Medicaid, etc. $15,000 per stay or a total of $800,000,000 billion per year most of whom die in the next year (556,000 die each year in nursing homes).

Need to Save $600 billion

The above definition puts a value of solving the health care problem to a necessity to reduce the wasted time, effort and loss of lives totaling 25% of the $2.5 trillion we are currently spending on ineffective results. Roughly $600,000,000,000 per year has to be saved now because the cascade is not only eating up resources it is bankrupting the American Society at the rate of $1,000,000,000,000 trillion per year due to the loss of productivity and competitiveness of the gross national product. We can no longer rationalize nor ration the country's resources on law makers that just add on 9,000 ear marks to an insane approach to Health Care Reform . . . we must stop all talk of throwing more money after bad . . . incremental change, coops, exchanges or a public option for further government control . . . that is true a health care fantasy and financial insanity.

If you think about it our health care costs are not only for services rendered but for those who make their salaries and do not produce a product . . . 19.7 million State and Federal government employees that cost us $1,100,000,000,000 trillion per year whose job it is to police the hundreds of thousands of laws heaped on businesses to control the bankers, the investors, the entrepreneurs and the voting public who want to believe we have a democracy and still cannot get their Senators or Representatives on the telephone to voice their opinion.

Jerry Rhoads

Health Care Deform (ity):

I could go on for pages about the rest of the problems in health care that the politicians do not want us to hear because they are part of the problem due to ineffective laws, regulations and payment formulas, the providers who are a part of the problem because they just want more money to waste, the employers who are a part of the problem because they only want out of the responsibility for the cost, the employees who are at fault and part of the problem because they take no responsibility for their own health and the cost of being unhealthy . . . so there lies the real problem. Every one of us needs to accept that there needs to be a dramatic paradigm shift from accepting illness and capitalizing on it to focusing on restoring health and preserving our resources, both monetary and human value.

The solution is simple, if we pay for illness not wellness, then let's reverse the logic . . . we talk of reforming a system of health care that is not standardized so it can be computerized . . . . we wish for better quality of life when we have not taken that as a priority when we eat and do not exercise for better fitness and health preservation habits . . . we all think that more money spent on poor results with less taxes (which does not add up) will make it better. Then why not pay for wellness . . . if Niagara Falls was going to flood New York City with its billions of gallons of water we would figure a way to reroute it so it does not kill 10 million people. How, we would turn off the faucet and change direction so we could control the cascading waters . . . so why not cascading health care costs . . . turn off the ineffective way we pay for illness and start paying for wellness (prevention, preservation and outcomes not just incomes).

All providers would be required to perform problem based diagnosis then have a plan for first preventing the problems then develop care plans that either alleviate the problems or prevent them through restorative models of care focused on the reduction of chronic diseases and develop rational strategies for improving the quality of life expectations for end of life services. We can use economic incentives to accomplish moral incentives . . . pay for outcomes not incomes . . . all providers would not get paid add on incentive payments unless they reduce the dependency of the patients on drugs, wheelchairs, re-hospitalizations, ER visits and alleviate the progression of chronic diseases.

We could then pay for the 50 million uninsured at the rate of $400 per month or $240,000,000,000 per year and still have money left for investing in prevention and health preservation natural methods to reduce poly pharmacy, diabetes and other chronic diseases.

Our academics who run health care call for evidenced based medicine and performance based payment but continue to use enforcement and art form health care guidelines that do not even follow the regulations and cannot be computerized or economized until there is ISO 12,000 standardization with six sigma type processes with the focus on preserving heath preventing chronic disease and paying for problem driven outcomes. Then we can have an integrated health care system that communicates the services among the providers and involves the patient and families in the pursuit of restorative services that put more of aging Americans back into community based programs.

FUNDING

Sounds great but how do we get from here to there. First we must take the onus of funding off the employer and taxpayer for universal health care. Yes all of us need to have coverage and a safety net but we all need to fund it as well. A withholding of before tax income for each individuals health care account can produce $3,000,000 over a work life at $400 per month compounded at 6% return when invested in the US economy.

With 160,000,000 million workers that produces
$718,000,000,000 per year in resources that would be deposited
into Mutual Health Insurance Company accounts (each American
can choose which company and is an shareholder in that company
and gets a potential return on the self-funded insurance health trust
(SHIFT of the paradigm) of $75,000,000,000 billion per year less
expenditures for each employee's self-directed health expenditures
for their chosen health care, fitness and nutrition options creating a
competitive market for their purchasing decisions.

The Mutual Health Insurance Companies investment of the
SHIFT savings accounts would be invested in the American
economy producing a dynamic emphasis on health enterprise
rather than a government controlled system that loses up to 50%
of the resources on payment for illness and ineffective regulations
and enforcement. The profits generated by the dynamic health
care investment program would produce an additional $1 trillion
dollars (based on interest income on investments, capital gains
and operating profits by the provider of health care services) in
additional tax income for State and Local Governments. America
then has solved the health care crisis and a sluggish economy
suffering from the Federal Reserve policies of a fatal attempt
to control inflation with a 500% increase in the Fed rate then
scrambling to cover it up with trillions of dollars of paper money.

SAFETY NETS

Medicare would be the safety net for catastrophic episodes for the
elderly.

Medicaid would be the coverage for the indigent unemployed.

Funding would continue to be out of the current methods . . .
withholding and social security trust funds. But the costs would

be cut by 80% with the funding during the employment period for long term care as well as hospitalization.

Self-Health thinking must come into our political system as well as our health care delivery system . . . with 77,000,000 million baby boomers aging at a frightful rate requires a dramatic change in thinking . . . treatment must become prevention and pills must become better nutrition and exercise, like it or not.

- So being healthy is a necessity to be attained

    — We are Born to be free from disease
    — We are Born to be a personal manager of our physic
    — We are Born to live long and productive lives
    — But we Live and Die by what we believe in and decide to be

- The privilege is earned by our good habits, positive thoughts and proactive living every day . . . it is our own recognition of the Red Zone and its dominance over our lives that create the will to be healthy, happy and prosperous!

John Stossel in his book "No, They Can't: Why Government Fails but Individuals Succeed" . . . government has become so bloated that practically every person in America is guilty of violating at least one of its arcane rules every day . . . the rules stem from the alphabet soup of government bureaucracy—IRS, DEA, EPA, OSHA, EEOC, TC, FDA—so government over regulation is what kills opportunity" not capitalism.

Jerry Rhoads

SHIFTING THE PARADIGM TO A SELF-HEALTH ENTERPRISE

Self-Health must be the responsibility of each individual to make a nationalized benefit package work . . . otherwise we will have a defined contribution plan with a defined benefit payment program being forced on the providers . . . that is more that socialized medicine . . . that is a Marxist formula for disaster because rationing based on age will occur with the elderly and disabled being put into end of life care tracks that are TRULY death panels.

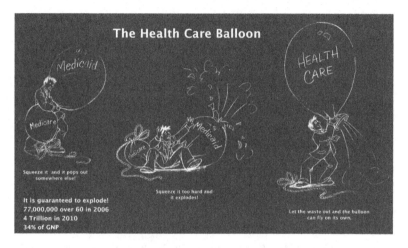

SELF-HEALTH DEFINED

You are the only one that can determine your life time . . . unless you get run over by a car . . . so the definition of Self-Health is the most important information you can receive:

S cience

E ngineered

L ife

F ulfillment

H ow you think determines your weight

E at when you are hungry and stop when you are full

A ge is not a factor to measure your longevity

L ife is your show and stage so act on it

T ime is a factor only in your use of it

H ealth is a journey not a destination

Healthy . . . Body . . . Mind . . . Heart . . . Soul = Self Health

Responsibility for one's own health will be the most important topic and initiative that will be enacted in the next decade because of the tsunami created by the birth rate of the Baby Boomers from 1945 to 1965.

BABY BOOMERS
BY JERRY RHOADS

The Boomers are coming
The impact is stunning
After the end of the Great war in '45
Brides and Grooms came alive

Boosting the pregnancy rate
Opening the baby gate
Christening 77 million by '65
Putting us in economic overdrive

Being the driving force of the Great Society
What they were promised is impropriety

However like much in today's politics
The Boomers will demand and vote for a fix

"Never fear The Boomers are here"

Chapter Four

Habits Control Lives

Red Zone Bad Habits

- Habits, good and bad, are stored in our Subconscious mind—who ever told us that our subconscious mind would determine our destiny? I learned this by looking for the reason I was not healthy, happy and prosperous. I found it in myself . . . in my decisions and values converted to a better life style.
- Consciously we live with the decisions we make but with little contemplation of the consequences. Those responses, according to the experts, become habits, good or bad, and do determine our health, happiness and prosperity. That is our value to ourselves.

Will, Willing and Willed
Jerry Rhoads

I can, I will, I am
To Make it Happen
I Can See the Vision
With Will to Understand

My Being is Willing
It to Happen
In the Future
By Instilling

The Habit
The Effort
The Routine
To Just Do It

No Amount of Fear
Can Overcome
My Will
To Endure

For I Have Been Willed
The Right
To Be Me
As Fear is Distilled

By My Seeing
That My Faith
To Be Me
Is More Then Doubt As my Being

Who would have thought that how we learned to function as a child would determine how long we will live, prosper and love our wife . . . it is all there in the subconscious shadows of our mind. Negative information from the time we are born, fed into our memory bank with no sense of urgency about its later affects.

Religions focus on cleansing our minds and souls but it is the heart that provides the feeling of what is wrong and what is right. It is the senses feeling the day to day occurrences that determine our future. So to ignore dreams, wishes, expectations and deny the wisdom of faith is a sorry situation to put yourself in . . . I know because it has taken me all these years to finally find my place in my heart.

The heart is the center of the solar system called humanity . . . without its sustenance we have no organs or mind. The blood flowing through our bodies have positive and negative molecules . . . these are dictated by the subconscious mind directives . . . it is impulsive and out of our real time control . . . it is a time bomb if left uncorrected from negative reactors to positive reactors.

Health Science and Psychology go hand in hand in understanding how our body and mind work but do not decide how our heart intercedes in day to day decisions we make for our response to subconscious brain washing. This is where a person's will must come into play in a decided effort to change the result of their actions. We call this breaking our bad habits. Good habits being those that warm the heart and connect us with other human beings.

Self-Health training programs: my daughter Kimber Leigh told me when I started my own business that I better stay healthy or starvation would likely be an outcome since I wouldn't have any imminent income if I weren't able to work. She suggested jumping rope since that was something she was learning how to do in high school gym class. It seemed like a good idea and I purchased a fairly cheap jump rope and for the next 4 years I jumped rope every morning . . . I started out only being able to do 10 reps, rest and do 100 in total . . . then I moved up to 100 reps, rest and do 1,000 in total . . . by the end of the 4 years I could jump an hour straight counting every rotation and got so I never missed . . . 10,000 reps each day 365 days per year = 3,650,000 reps per year for 4 years or 14 million 600 hundred thousand repetitions.

Did this put me in the Self-Health Zone . . . no because I did not concern myself with what I was eating . . . omelet's, bacon, red meat, sodium, saturated fat, etc. Then I read the Diamond's book "Fit for Life" and it changed my thinking to exercising my mouth and stomach as well as my body. Life style issues are as important in Self-Health exercise as are the physical attributes.

Not only did I change my eating habits, I changed my mode of exercise from the repetitive boredom of rope jumping to the more stimulating aerobic exercise called jogging . . . which evolved into competitive running . . . always trying to better the distance and time of the previous day . . . 7 days per week, 7 miles per day on the same route for 7 years is what my running career evolved into. 17,885 miles later injuries set in and plantar factitious forced me to the bicycle. That led to a stationary bike that lasted 4 years and I went back to running every day, 7 days per week but varied the distance and route. So for some twenty years I focused on one exercise every day . . . did not take a day off and never missed any work. But was I in the Red Zone mentally and thinking but in the Self-Health physically? Yes . . . I was not mentally healthy.

During this time my business was a roller coaster of risk taking, successful growth but unsustainable business plan and a bankruptcy followed . . . leaving me with a strong endurance and a weak mind. The exercise went to weight training to prove how much I could do and some cross training with aerobic exercise devices filling in . . . over those years before and after the business failure I always played tennis competitively and attained a 4.5 ranking playing leagues and local tournaments. It was all about ego not about wellness, fitness and full body and mental Self-Health habits.

I finally moved out of the Red Zone when my wife of 54 years and I decided we needed to connect in some exercise program and started walking and roller blading together. We walked, talked and bladed holding hands. We got so we could walk 9 miles and roller blade 12 miles without stopping . . . and found this allowed us to bond by talking and not just sitting and looking at each other over a meal and sleeping through a movie. This is true Self-Health activity and it is easy . . . walking shoes, a safe long trail, good weather and a commitment to just doing it. We now walk at least once a week on Saturday together, I work out on cross training every morning but Monday and she is doing yoga and palates once to twice per week.

Sex, Kids and Rock & Roll—Dancing our way into the Self-Health

Shari Rhoads and I are blessed with our health, happiness and prosperity because of our life style. We met in High School, she a freshman and I a sophomore. Two years before I spotted this new girl standing in front of the Junior High Building talking to another seventh grader. That was in 1953 and evolved into 54 years of marriage with 4 grown children, 12 grandchildren and a new great grandson. We have avoided the red zone and attract Self-Health habits . . . our parents died early deaths in nursing homes and did not have the opportunities we have had. We have not retired and plan not to. We have worked together since 1992 in the health care field.

Prior to that I started my health care career in 1962 auditing Blue Cross hospitals and was on the team that rolled out Medicare for Blue Cross in hospitals and nursing homes. My specialty is Medicare and Medicaid rules and regulations that the government rarely follows. CMS the paying agent decides what not to pay using intimidation and illegal guidelines depriving the seniors their skilled nursing benefits, and has since 1975. If you doubt this fact pull up Federal Court Cases Fox v Bowne 1986, and Jimmo v Sibuleus, 2012 that found that the government has been misinterpreting Medicare for 30 years.

Shari is going to be 74 in October and I will be 75 in November 2014 . . . our pictures in Part II are proof that this personal diary of why life styles and habits determine longevity, prevention of illness and preservation of self-worth. Our lives have attracted not only each other but successes in our businesses and raising a great family. We have always been in love and love to dance . . . our children are all artistic and we believe in the arts. And when we are asked our secret I slyly say "sex, kids and rock and roll" because it is true. When we go on a cruise to celebrate our wedding anniversary we go to the dance floor rather than the slot machines and only eat when we are hungry, only eat what is healthy and stop when we are full. Shari weighs in at 112 and I at 180 . . . she has taken Dr. Oz's biological aging test and scores out at 54, due to her pacemaker inserted to fix a congenital arrhythmia and I at 52. Our expectation are to live past 100 and never look back.

Why is this important. Well if you are writing a book on health and health care it assumed that you have to be a doctor or PhD or some government official . . . well Shari and I are neither. We just have found the fountain of youth and it is in all of us . . . it is in our minds if we develop that part of the brain that holds our subconscious habits. Is it possible to replace bad physical and mental habits. Of course it is if you are motivated to live better longer. I have written a series of Self-Health books that focus on your brain not your body . . . because your mind will correct the condition of your body if you let it. If you doubt this go to the Self-Health cultures and look at what makes them different from us Red Zone Americans. That is what this book is about, and how the health care industry can convert from a pursuit of treatment and prescriptions to a pursuit of wellness of mind first and body second.

Our children . . . and we have four ranging in age from 42 to 52 have their own wellness and fitness routines using Self-Health activities . . . mostly with our 12 grandchildren who are into sports, dancing, cheerleading, boating, fishing, hunting and loving the Self-Health . . . although there are Red Zone influences in pursuit of them they manage to keep a happy balance with the video games, Facebook, I-phones, I-pads and all the other texting-entertainment devices.

THE FOUNTAIN OF YOUTH

Clearly most people blame circumstances for bad luck and avoidance of being diligent about their personal health. But Shari and I believe we have found the six steps to the Fountain of Youth:

1. Love
2. Family and friends
3. Work and play
4. Happiness
5. Regular Sexual encounters
6. Regular physical exercise

As you notice there is no mention of diets, depriving yourself of food, including your favorites, money, retirement, more time off, fasting, counting calories or group activities. In our experience these take care of themselves if you practice self-health thinking . . . just look at the results as you change your subconscious habits.

For example Shari and Jerry Rhoads have taken the Real Age test and have 54 years and 52 years as their biological age versus their chronological ages of 73 and 74. Life can and should begin at seventy.

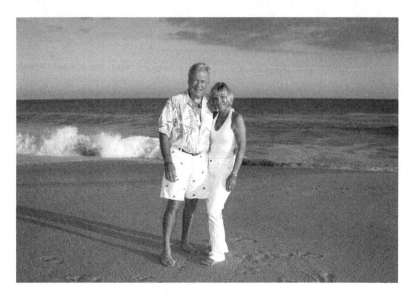

BABY BOOMERS

Starting in 2005 they want to retire
Long before they expire
Maxing out their social security checks
Leaving entitlements as fiscal wrecks

Paying their share of tax bills if wealthy
Believing that Medicare will keep them healthy
Being the driving force of the Great Society
What they were promised is impropriety

Chapter Five

Thoughts Control Habits

Red Zone Thoughts

- Can we be healthy by thinking that we want to be healthy? Yes, we usually get what we want if we truly want it bad enough to take action.
- Thoughts are the beginning of everything in our world, but it is action that determines what we get.
- So mental exercising is as important as physical exercising. Science is proving that active minds live longer than dullards.
- We become what and who we think we are . . . not what we were but what we think and believe we can be.

We have so long failed to understand the wonderful power of thought for it is taught by every religion and philosophy in the history of the world. Paul, when in captivity and chained to a Roman soldier gave to the world this message:

> *Finally, brethren whatsoever things are true, whatsoever things are honest, whatsoever things are just, whatsoever things are pure, whatsoever things are lovely and of good report; if there be any virtue and there be any praise, think on these things.*

Most of us have overlooked the meaning of that verse. We have been so busy admiring its beauty of diction that we failed to place emphasis on the word think. If everybody followed Paul's injunction and thought only in terms of truth, honesty, justice, purity and loveliness, this world would be transformed from a planet of confusion, sickness and poverty into one of radiant health, happiness, and prosperity.

Quoted from Venice Bloodworth's wonderful book The Key to Yourself.

If we follow our conscious minds we will never find true happiness due to acquired habits and attitudes . . . so Self-Health starts with the subconscious mind by stop thinking about failure and start controlling your thoughts through mental exercises that will enable you to accept and enjoy physical exercises . . . these are called affirmations and confirmations stated to yourself in the quiet times . . . when these thoughts become the habit you will find guilt only in the habit of putting them off. "I do not love working out I only feel fulfilled by the act of doing it" . . . Jack Lalanne . . . the Godfather of Fitness" who lived healthy, happy and prosperous until he was 96.

For a quick reminder just think the 4 w's, who, what, when, where for the first step to self health: who is you, what is your mind, when is now and where is in your own home. Self-Health does not require an exotic gym or setting. Much of my mental exercises are done in bed before I get up in the morning. My weakness mental control is when I wake up worrying about the past not planning the future. Many times I have to remind myself that 85% of what I worry about never happens and the other 15% is only half as bad as it seems . . . why should I ruin my day, week and life on 7.5% of my induced worries. My time is much better spent envisioning how I will be happy, health and prosperous.

Much of religion teaches the very exercises that are proposed in my Self-Health formula. Prayer is envisioning better times and hope . . . hope is the best way to get in an "I Can" mood . . . a good mood is the start of the "I Will" action . . . action is the way to make your future that you envision to stay positive . . . staying positive will put you out front of your life . . . being in front of your life proves that Self-Health works. So, good luck in working on your most valuable asset . . . your mind . . . that will inspire you to work on your body.

Will this quickly and forever change your outlook, personality, values and ethics . . . no . . . it requires a daily, weekly, monthly, yearly and life long commitment to improving your self worth . . . this is what creates the changes that you yourself want. It takes work.

MENTAL EXERCISING

(Stop negative thinking use mental exercises, start feeling good)

Thoughts are things. Your current situation is a result of your thinking, not your circumstances. The experts on behaviors all agree we are what we think we are. But we are what our thinking habits are. If we want to change our thoughts we must CHOOSE to change our thought processes . . . most of which are learned from childhood and have become responses to situations not well thought out consequences.

What is mental exercising? Generally speaking we learn by repetition . . . so by reading and rereading the mental exercises in this book hopefully will start you thinking and acting in a different way. We have been taught, in most instances, what not to do . . . not what to do. That flaws our results. Now we must turn the tables and concentrate on what to do.

There is a story told in baseball about Yogi Berra when he was the skipper for the New York Yankees . . . in the ninth inning of game 7 of the World Series the opposition had the tying run on base and two outs . . . Yogi goes to the mound to direct the relief pitcher on what to do . . . he proceeded to tell the pitcher "to not throw the ball over the plate" . . . walked back to the dugout and watched the pitcher do exactly what was planted in his head . . . he threw the ball over the plate and the hitter drove it into the seats to win the game.

Yogi was great catcher but not a successful manager . . . instead of telling the pitcher what to do; "throw the ball outside or inside" he planted a seed of failure in the pitcher's head that created a negative outcome.

What to do is being conscious of our decisions and not letting our subconscious control our lives . . . for it is the subconscious that plays back learned responses based on "what not to do".

You can have a choice if you reprogram responses. So, to change the way we respond to situations not circumstances we must change our subconscious. This will take mental exercising our daily activities in advance in a positive manner.

For example: today is Monday and we have just had a miserable weekend due to anger and disappointment. The mental state is one of dread and dislike for our jobs and current circumstances. The mental state is negative and the day will be negative if approached from this perspective. When this happens awareness must enter into your mind and take a 180 degree turn for the betterment of your day. So on Monday you will want to forget Saturday and Sunday . . . then knowingly basing the week on better thoughts for better days.

Better thoughts (practice exercises):

- I am happy NOW
- I am healthy NOW
- I am a better person NOW

- I am successful NOW
- I am strong NOW
- I am stress free NOW

Better results (Monday evening):

- I could have been happier today because of

  _____

- I could have been healthier today because of

  _____

- I could have had a better attitude today because of

  _____

- I could have been more successful today because of

  _____

- I could have been stronger today because of

  _____

- I could have been stress free today if I would have

  _____

Better Tomorrow: (repeat the exercises daily or at least weekly and you will be amazed how you improve your stress free aging results). However, on Sunday I cannot make up for Monday through Friday indiscretions just through church and prayer. One day of advent cannot make up for 6 days of decent. Lives are gained or lost on religion when it is the life style and heart strings that determine our spirituality. To be good is to be good on Monday through Sunday with our actions and reactions to self-control and self—affirmations. Our body is our pulpit, our mind is our word, our heart is our haven, our deeds are our tithes, and our spirit is our heaven on earth.

CHAPTER SIX

Actions Control Fate

Red Zone Actions

- Is life circumstantial and happenstance with little under our control? Or is it our decisions and actions that determine circumstances and what happens to us?
- It can be either . . . you have to determine what your life's outcomes are or let your habits dictate the end result based on your subconscious mind's memory responses using past out dated data. Our computer brain retrieves the negative spam as well as the few positive emails.

NEGATIVE SITUATIONS

In reading Self-Help books for the last 37 years since I started my own business I have found a way to activate positive thinking to overcome a childhood of negative re-enforcement from my parents. They were a product of the great depression and were brought up in survival environment and with little to hope for. My mother lived in a log cabin in Missouri until she married my father and moved to a farm in Iowa. My father was brought up on a farm in Iowa and took to the rails as a hobo during the late 1920's with two of his brothers.

So at the age of 18 he was traveling all over the country riding railroad cars with other misplaced and hungry souls. His and other stories have been captured on a program done by the National Enquirer magazine. His story was documented as a day worker who got $1 per day for working 10 hours in the fields picking corn and bailing hay and maybe getting a free meal at noon time. This lasted 4 years until they could return to the farm that had seeds for planting and harvesting. His home life was fairly stable with 5 brothers and 2 sisters who all farmed then moved into to town and worked in factories in Des Moines.

My mother on the other hand had the life of poor dirt farmers with little food and no money. She, her brother and sister were the victims of physical and mental abuse that affected her the rest of her life. Due to their home life her brother was a deserter from the Army, and a sexual abuser of his own children, nieces and others in his life shortened by cancer. Her sister was also in an abusive marriage that resulted in her husband and son committing suicide.

I am sure if researched they lived interesting but Red Zone lives without much of a desire or life style of good nutrition and fitness activities. It was more where is the next meal coming from without concern for its content . . . everyone in those days were under weight and obesity was only demonstrated at the County Fair on the Mid-Way by the Fat Lady.

SELF-HEALTH
END ZONE POSITIVE ACTIONS

(Stop hating your job, sports team, financial situation by using this book to do creative positive action for happiness, start loving your life)

The power of positive thinking makes common sense but uncommon among most Americans. We are buried in negativism . . . newspapers, tabloids, television cruelty, movie perversions, gangster rap, violent reality shows, aberrant sexual behaviors, etc, etc,

The world is negative because we tend to see things in a fearful way. We by nature fear the future because of the unknowns. Our own world does not have to be negative but our subconscious has been filled with negativity. To overcome this situation takes acknowledging its existence and a concerted effort to reprogram our subconscious.

How is that possible when we continue to respond when we are confronted by crisis, stress, cynical thoughts, fear, anger, sexual thoughts, false hopes, failures, fantasies, lost dreams, etc, etc,

In my case much of my negative thoughts were about the fear of rejection and being incapable to control my emotions. Success was a pursuit not a result of preparation and dedication. However, they existed from a childhood of little love, support or encouragement . . . my parents were a product their fears, habits and rejections.

Then came LOVE into my life.

- L ife
- O ccurs
- V irtually
- E very way

When I found sports I found a way to feel good about my talents . . . I was good at it . . . not excellent but better than most . . . however, I was never the star . . . just the backup or the sixth man. But I had this drive, desire to be the best . . . which spurred me on to this day. I loved it.

Then came a business career that was not much more than reactionary. I did very well in school, particularly college but still was not the 4 pointer or the magna cum lade. I was rewarded the highest business award in college. I loved it.

My marriage was very positive and filled the blanks for my lack of love and support from my parents . . . our children were healthy, happy and thrived on my attitude that "can't never did anything" and dreams were to be pursued not squelched. I loved it.

My wife and son helped me form a better business after an initial set back. We now are building for the future to assist the elderly to be healthy and have facilities where we are providing restorative services to overcome the bad habits of everyone's earlier years. I love it.

Even though most of my life has resulted in positive results I still feel unfulfilled. Why? Because negativity still lurks in my subconscious . . . I work daily on suppressing the darkness and focusing on the bright lights of tomorrow. Today has already been set in the stone of my past thoughts and actions . . . no changing that . . . but the next day (s) are up to me and my ability to think positively in a negative world. Still I love the challenge.

I get mad at the Cubs and the Bears, I rant at the politicians, I wonder about money, I hope for attainment of my goals, I fear the unknown, I am a victim of mood swings . . . I certainly have my negative moments . . . but my study continues on how to keep a positive outlook that results in positive outcomes . . . I read Deepak Chopra, almost daily, I read the Secret at least once a week, I read "The Key To Yourself" as well . . . I work at it. Still I love the Cubs and Bears.

But probably more important I believe I can change my attitude and future if it becomes negative by saying "remember" if you start out negative you will finish the day negative so why would you do it that way . . . and it always works out that the day is dependent on my every morning thinking not just my doing. Just speaking the word love puts you in a positive state of mind.

The next most important function in my daily routine is some form of physical exercise . . . distance running (an obsessive 7 miles a day, 7 days per week, 52 weeks per year for 7 years), rope jumping (obsessively counted reps and could jump for an hour without stopping . . . 10,000 reps) cycling when I injured my heel from plantar factitious, a lifting weights until I injured my diaphragm, cardio on stair stepper, elliptical, tread mill, and finally fairly good tennis player/frustrated athlete. All of this was more for keeping my head straight than my physic. I hate the work and love the results.

I never have and never will tell my children or you that you have to exercise to be happy and healthy and prosperous but I am here to testify that any semblance of success I have had and the fact that I am now 74 years old, have been married 54years to the same great woman (who looks 50 at the age of 73), did 74 pushups for my 4 children and 12 grandchildren and started a new business at the age of 70 are more a product of mental and physical exercise than sheer talent. I love being fit.

Just to let you know I plan to do 80 pushups when I am 80, 90 when I am 90 and 100 when I am 100 . . . after that I plan to slow down. In the next life it is all mental anyway!

Self-Help books have been an important part of my life . . . early on I was into Earle Nightengale, then Napoleon Hill, now it is The Secret, Depok Chopra and human psychology. They all carry the same message: you are what you think you are . . . you become what you want to be . . . but random conditioning of your subconscious mind relegates you to your past.

This SELF-HEALTH BOOK forces the issue of moving your thinking in a different path so the future does a mental house cleaning and a new thought conditioning called "I am happy, healthy and prosperous" affirmation enough to replace the subconscious feelings for negativity programmed into all of us by parents, media and life's problems and challenges.

For me mental and physical exercise have enable me to overcome a negative self-image, a fear of the unknown, because I now can control my thoughts about what I want and it will appear as it has for many others.

CHAPTER SEVEN

Earning Self-Health Privileges

In the following chapters we will focus on **WHAT MATTERS** and how to change your paradigm from the Red Zone to End Zone life style by understanding the negative effects of a Red Zone World.

Move **A**head **T**hinking **T**hat **E**arning **E**nergy **R**everses **S**ins of the past . . . Because What You Don't Want Destroys Thoughts of What You Do Want. So focus on turning dreams on with meditation about what you want until it appears.

Thinking in the Red Zone is best defined by our Tabloid media that uses disasters, failures, bad news and bad weather to get our attention then proceeds to bring in positive factors as the end of the entertainment product. Unfortunately, the endings are not usually happy but a sad rendition of those lives that will continue to be lived in the Red Zone . . . Brittney Spears, Lady Gaga, Elvis, Mike Tyson, Lindsey Lohan, Whitney Houston, etc. Lives, that were, or will be, shortened by their Red Zone habits.

Is it really fair to single out the celebrities . . . no probably not . . . look around 60% of Americans are obese and 35% morbidly so. Most are not physically toned or make any effort to improve their physical, mental and emotional wellbeing. Am I being judgmental or just trying to sell a book on Self-Health? Probably both . . . and it seems self-serving to brag about my own fitness or health condition but the intention is to alert those that are aging that we all owe it to one another to aspire for better health so we can afford other endeavors . . . 80% of the current health care dollar is spent on illness not on keeping well or fit.

The Government in all its wisdom currently only pays for treatment, hospital tests and prescription drugs for chronic diseases and the elderly has 4 to 5 each. There are no active programs for any of us, except the wealthy who can have personal trainers that pays for prevention of chronic diseases or preservation of personal health to enable us all to live longer and more productive lives. We are all victims of a socialized approach to medicine and a institutionalized mentality for dealing with illness. But the enemy is not the Government it is the voters who continue to put them back in office and not holding them accountable in the way the money is spent . . . expediency is their thinking because they do not have the sufficient resources to prevent and preserve health that the have not's deal with daily.

Basically we need a Self-Health approach to public service . . . everyone needs to commit some of their careers and time to participating in Government, as the founding fathers had envisioned. Currently the Red Zone negative effects are destroying our stature and standing in the world.

- Imbalance of trade
- Declining value of our dollar
- Unsustainable deficits in our national equity due to unfathomable debt
- Lowering levels of our Gross National and Domestic Products and our World economic influence
- Wavering strength of our consumers due to unemployment and exorbitant taxation at all levels of our State, Federal and local Governments
- Unrealistic pensions for Government officials triggered by unionization
- Uncontrollable cost of energy and labor
- Trillions of dollars of our economy spent on weapons of mass destruction, under the guise of National Defense, with no amounts being spent on peace making infra structures . . . just foreign aide that has no fiscal or social accountability.
- Governments that are dominated by attorneys and lawmakers who do not know how to create jobs and sustain the American Enterprise System.

Our National Leaders are imbibing the wind not sustaining it . . . third generation politicians who have never had to meet a payroll or miss a meal are making decisions to perpetuate their personal stature and standing not America's.

BABY BOOMERS
BY JERRY RHOADS

Being the driving force of the Great Society
What they were promised is impropriety
However like much in today's politics
The Boomers will demand and vote for a fix
"Never fear The Boomers are here"

CHAPTER EIGHT

What You Think Matters

- Thinking is hard work if you want to control it . . . bad habits from the subconscious get in the way.
- Reprogramming your subconscious is very hard work . . . cleansing all that negative data that is in your memory bank.
- Accepting things the way they are is the easy way out . . . determining the way you want them to be is a process of reprogramming your responses to situations, plans and relationships.
- Your health, happiness and prosperity depend on it, so does the Self-Health commitment.
- Thinking will provide the direction and motivation to change your Red Zone habits to Self-Health habits.

MASTER OF GOOD HABITS

(Stop destructive habits that age you by using this book to form good habits, learn how to control the subconscious impulses day by day listening to your own affirmations . . . ideas and thoughts then create your world)

Captain of myself made state, Master of my fate. Am I really in control of my destiny? Or is it some supreme being that has me on a puppet string? It is whatever you decide . . . you are master of your thoughts if you decide to be and then you are captain of your fate. Destiny is never fixed and circumstances are determined by the past . . . so invest today wisely since it will determine where you are tomorrow. Your mental capacity is unlimited (President JFK had an ordinary IQ and an extraordinary EQ . . . so may you).

We started out speaking of good habits and have spent most chapters on that topic . . . the topic of you. YOU are the center of your world, your universe, your future . . . that is the exciting knowledge that I have learned through hours upon hours of reading and thinking and meditating about. Fear drove me most of the time:

- Fear of failure
- Fear of not being able to pay my bills
- Fear of not being accepted (rejection)
- Fear of dying early
- Fear of living less
- Fear of the fear itself

I succeeded in squelching the fear through mental and physical exercises. I am not saying "if I can do it you can" that is condescending at the very least . . . I am encouraging you to overcome fear by changing how you think about yourself. This takes changing your routines, your habits, your actions, your future by changing your NOW . . . the past is gone and needs to be buried because that is not you NOW.

Pick a book . . . it is not a come down to find the answers in knowledge or GOOD WILL HUNTING adventures. It is reeducating your subconscious to be what you want to be . . . want is the main ingredient . . . not money . . . not talent . . . not relationships . . . not love . . . those are results of you exercising your right to want, give and receive your desires, your dreams, your goals.

Being a master at anything takes according to Malcolm Gladwell a minimum of 10,000 hours (5 continuous years) of training and preparation . . . athletes, scientists, performers, politicians, attorneys, business entrepreneurs, physicians if they are any good at all have to study and go into a timeless obsession to be the best at something and then they are what they are. You are what you expect to be and want to be . . . master your good habits, be not your bad habits, by being stress free from doubt:

- Decide that you can overcome your fears . . . state them then confront them
- Set simple goals that can be accomplished then savor more ambitious successes
- Find a place for yourself satisfaction in giving to others and loving your present life
- Prepare each day with a healthy agenda (age-nda means a health plan for the day including food, exercise, thoughts of love, acts of kindness)
- Stick your neck out for causes you stand for then the take action to help others find their agenda

No matter how many books are written on self-help or self-engineering none can be complete without putting the most important ingredient first . . . that is the commitment to family . . . to marriage regardless of sexual orientation . . . to offspring and to wellspring. Yes commitment; not let's try and see if it works . . . it will work if you work for it . . . divorce is the most destructive force we have in America for negativity, loss of health, loss of wealth, loss of dignity and loss of our children's future. Yes commitment to one's responsibility to self and others is the science of Self-Health.

No I am not foolish enough to say every marriage is going to work . . . that is not realistic . . . however, that is not a bad idea for most who want happiness, health and prosperity. Otherwise the reverse typically results . . . unhappiness, unhealthiness and financial setbacks

SELF—WORTH CAPITAL

(Stop being angry with yourself by using this book to see yourself-worth, start feeling good, thinking well and being healthy)

Over the ages man has asked man what am I worth . . . never realizing that worth is determined by one's self not those around us. When we are worthy we attract more worth until we are wealthy.

Why do we ask others when the answer is usually couched in what the other person thinks of themselves . . . if they are unhappy with themselves we will not and can not get any positive feedback from them . . . if they are happy with themselves they don't want to make it any easier for you then they had it . . . so guess what . . . the truth is in the ears of the listener not in the voice of the speaker. You make your own self-worth minute by minute, hour by hour, day by day.

The saying is "mental attitude has more to do with success than mental capacity" . . . if you want it bad enough it shall be yours. But most people do look outside themselves for encouragement, fulfillment, love, understanding, support, faith, endearment, etc. etc. Do they find it there? That is the question that we need to answer.

Who is your best friend? Does he or she really know all your thoughts about them and yourself? If they did they would not be your friend. We do not live out our thoughts . . . we hide behind them and rationalize them so we do not offend others nor expose ourselves. Most of those thoughts are negative due to a lack of recognition and cognition that we are what we think we are.

To build our self-net-worth we need to invest our self-worth capital in developing knowledge, faith, love, loyalty, honesty, commitment, expectations on what is right for others as well as ourselves. The beggar is repulsive and rejected because we see ourselves in them and fear those consequences of bad luck and avoid feeling good about our own good luck. By giving to the beggar we can feel good about our good luck regardless of how the money is used. True Giving opens the heart not the pocketbook . . . if it is about affording a gift it is not a gift it is a sacrifice and that does not build self-worth it erodes self-respect.

Can we give enough to feel good about ourselves? Most times the act is for reason other than being good to others. Americans during this depressed economy are withdrawing into themselves to protect their pride and livelihood. This is the time we can reap the most from our giving because there are always those that are worse off . . . the very act will make our value increase in our heart and leave the payment of bills to our head. We then will have more coming than going by doing good. This is not just a religious concept it is the Law of Attraction at work again . . . good attracts good . . . need generates a use of our talents . . . demand for our talents increases our net self-worth. That is what generates dollars and makes human value into capital for our children and grandchildren.

The free enterprise concept of the Law of Attraction is bankruptcy which is America's willingness to allow us to fail then rekindle our fire and do what our dreams want us to do . . . yes it is 100% mental . . . everything starts with an idea, a thought and a vision . . . you can be either the envision(er) or the envision(ee) but the point is you decide. Either way you are allowed to fail then reorganize and succeed . . . no other economic system allows for this. This is the greatest part of capitalism versus the other isms . . . we are allowed to freely choose to fail then choose to succeed . . . just remember it is all founded on how you think and who you want to be.

BABY BOOMERS
BY JERRY RHOADS

However like much in today's politics
The Boomers will demand and vote for a fix
Finding no equity in money-tics
Like the ride of Paul Revere
"Never fear The Boomers are here"

CHAPTER NINE

What You Do Matters

- Our daily routines are what get us in trouble . . . we put off the important actions for the easy ones.
- Have you noticed that work is boring if we continue to only do the easy things first . . . the hard ones are what separate us from the Red Zone pack.
- So doing is to list the things you want to change in pursuing health, happiness and prosperity . . . then do them first and foremost every day.
- Example: how hard is it to walk a mile . . . not very hard unless you decide you don't have the time or need to. Hard is in the mind of the RED ZONER . . . as Nike says just do it until it is a habit.
- The trip from Red Zone to the Self-Health Zone is entirely up to you based on your daily decisions and activities.

FINDING GOOD

(Stop finding fault with others by using this book to find good in everyone, start finding more friends)

GOOD WILL HUNTING was a successful film, story and won Oscars for Matt Damon and Ben Affleck and turned their lives around. The messages that the film portrayed are meaningful to all of us . . . we all have a God Given Talent that needs expression . . . if you do not express it you will suffer the frustration of being unfulfilled.

From that film the word "Karma" comes to mind which is your good will planting of the seeds of self-worth and "Dharma" which is your good will finding and harvesting the good in your life. We then can be truly happy, healthy and prosperous in our daily LIFE.

America is addicted to athletes and celebrities to the extent that they become folk heroes without usually earning the role. We find out later that they are just ordinary people doing extra ordinary things because they believe they can. That is the reason I kept reminding my children to pursue their dreams and that "can't never did anything" and "can discovered America and Americans discovered GOOD WILL HUNTING.

Will Hunting was wasting his talent on being one of the boys in the hood but was a genius mathematician who would never have been discovered if Robin Williams had not took him by the head and straightened him into a wonderful success story. Who will be your mentor . . . have you found one yet. They are out there waiting for you to want to be good enough to think and grow rich. This is call the Law of Attraction . . . likes attract likes.

Well you have to be looking or have opportunity take you there because most of us do not have the awareness to recognize our special talents let alone capitalize on them. In my case I went from being a bored auditor to becoming a health care expert because the company I worked for said I could, and would not accept anything less. But my first mentor was a rabbi who owned nursing homes and he spotted my talent . . . knowledge about the Medicare programs and enlisted my expertise in his businesses . . . he let me practice on his playground and he paid me for it.

After taking on his facilities and turning them around I worked myself out of a job at the age of 45, and met my next mentor who had responsibilities for 50 long term care facilities and I was hired as a consultant to turn-a-round the worst of the worst. I again worked myself out of a job and at the age of 47 went back into my own business.

I found these two gentlemen who believed in me and my talent . . . it then inspired me to take on a new business at the age of 70 to practice what I have learned so I can help the elderly and disabled have a quality of life . . . extend their lives not just end them.

My wife and son are my partners and we are committed to finding a good way to manage the aging process for ourselves and our patients. And through the Law of Attraction (likes attract likes) we plan to build a franchise business that will serve aging Americans in a positive and stimulating environment.

Looking back I feel I was destined to find good expression of my talents because my first memories of the elderly was a rest home across from my house in Indianola, Iowa . . . these poor souls were spending all day in rocking chairs with nothing to do or live for . . . to me that seemed wrong and it still does. And now I can do something about it.

The D. C. Whitehouse (named after Shari's mother Dorotha Corny White) is our dream house dedicated to changing the lives of aging America through better life actions through planning and pre-forming attitudes about age. We need to become a nation of health preservers not life preservers . . . this all starts in our home with our children and their habits . . . ironically their habits are your habits . . . like it or not the future of our children is set in motion by our feelings and actions about ourselves. The ripple effect of you becoming happy, healthy and prosperous is amazing for the future of your children but America in general.

CHAPTER TEN

What You Consume Matters

- Is obesity a problem in the world today? Oh yeah it is . . . because we all eat to feed our insecurities not our minds or bodies.
- I read a book recently that gave the best advice ever . . . eat when you are hungry . . . stop when you're full . . . eat what you enjoy and the pounds will take care of themselves.
- Nonsense . . . we must suffer to be thin . . . oh yeah is it working for you that way . . . try the advice . . . it works in the Self-Health Zone.
- Can we consume our way to happiness and better outcomes . . . no that is Red Zone thinking.
- Consuming the chemicals we are taking into our bodies is creating the very diseases we are fighting.
- Nature rejects chemicals and so does our immune system until it is overwhelmed by senseless consumption.

AGELESS DIET

(Stop eating whatever you desire and use this book to plan your ageless diet, start eating for joy)

Our eating habits are also inherited from our past conditioning. Good habits are not the typical pattern of growing up with parents who have bad eating habits. So we have to reprogram our eating habits if we want to; Never be Too Old To LIVE.

I am not one to preach but would like to teach you what I have learned about eating. If it is artificially tasty it is probably not good for you. For instance fast foods, which take the brunt of the bad habits we form, are flavored for instant gratification . . . not permanent health.

Okay this is just common knowledge and sense . . . so how do I break these bad eating habits so I am aging slower and more rewardingly. The fact is I won't live forever, so why shouldn't I just enjoy it and move on. Try being the Biggest User of this book and not the Biggest Loser of this LIFE!

Facts:

- 65% to 70% of Americans are obese or on their way
- 80% of Americans will die before their time
- 90% of Americans do not knowingly strive to live for wellness and fitness
- 100% of Americans eventually die but most due to untimely deaths (always too Young to Die)
- I for one do not want to die before my time, and my time is under my control

I am not going to give you a recipe for what you should eat . . . you know it already . . . we all have it in front of us daily and we just ignore the facts. We want to be satisfied rather than healthy, happy and prosperous. Why because we think our poor health is circumstantial instead of self-inflicted desires to satisfy taste not pursuit of Self-Health health.

But what you can do is this:

- Be conscious of what you are eating go to <u>www.drfuhrman</u>.com/ *consult Dr. Fuhrman's micronutrient plan and find your best diet.*
- Look at the labels and plan a better approach to consumption **www.realage.com** *Dr. Oz and Dr. Roizen guide you to better intake and the impact it has on aging.*
- At least eat one good meal per day, then two per day, then three . . . a progression is better then no improvement at all *<u>www.livestrong.com</u>* **Harvey and Marilyn Diamond Fit for Life formula takes us to the eating habits to change your weight and quality of life.**
- Keep off the scale and make the reason for healthy eating your age not your weight **www.hubs.com/Venice-Bloodworth** *and read Dr. Bloodworth's book* **Key to Yourself** *for the mind to direct the body's consumption in its journey to the Self-Health.*

A good indicator of your results will be your natural weight, your best energy level, your improved strength, your improved skin and muscle tone, your improved feeling of self—worth . . . is it worth it . . . try it. Feeding the body the right nutrients is the quickest route for our spirit to cleanse our soul as well as our pipes.

Eating for longevity is a new concept in an old thinking world. Conventional wisdom has dumbed down America to think that consumption is the American Dream. While common sense is numbed down with drugs, alcohol, sugar, salt, fats delivered to us faster and faster. In the olden days consumption was based on earning power not credit power. Our credit card crack is burying us in debt and fat cells. Consumption is the nightmare instead of the dream of longevity, prosperity and happiness. To reverse this red zone culture takes individual commitment:

1. I will take my consumption seriously with a plan.

2. I will move from the red zone to the Self-Health thinking.
3. I will assist others in doing the same.
4. I will do my part to change the American nightmare to a dream of living longer, and better.
5. I will find hope and happiness in my physic and my personal beauty.
6. I will never fall backwards and will always commit to move forwards influencing my offspring to pursue health not just wealth.
7. I will realize that the red zone is an individual fault not a national campaign and the Self-Health Zone is my personal journey to longevity, prosperity and happiness.

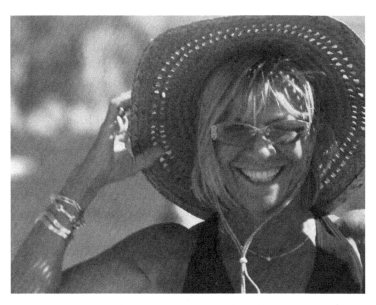

Can you believe this person is 70 in this picture . . . SHE IS NOW 73 (see pictures in Part II of this book) and looks 50 and acts 40 and feels 30 and outlives 20 others her age . . . AGELESS WITH THAT SMILE . . . She is picky about what she eats, only eats when she is hungry, eats what she likes and stops before she is full. (WEIGHT 112) . . . like her Aunt Edith and her Mother Dorotha.

A TRUE MIRACLE AND SHE JUST HAPPENS TO BE MY WIFE OF 54 YEARS.

She is like her MOTHER WHO DIED PREMATURELY AT 92 and her Aunt Edith who lived to be a ripe ole 109 outliving her husband Ernie who preceded her in death at 101. THEIR FAVORITE FOODS WERE THOSE PRODUCED ON THE FARMS and were not continually fighting chronic diseases the way we do now with pills and chemicals by preventing them with COD LIVER OIL and ben-gay. Their life style of work and healthy eating contributed to better family relationships, fewer divorces and better social mores.

Just because we live longer now, does not justify the deterioration of the American health profile . . . we live longer not because of pills and technology . . . it is we do not have to perform physical work the way our fore fathers were subjected to . . . convenience and ease of physical life is killing our immune system so we need a certain level of physical activity to support our nutritional health.

DEATH BY BELT SIZE

A study indicates that kidney disease patients with larger waists also have a higher risk of death. Researchers saw it in four years of data on about 5,800 kidney disease patients. At Loyola University Health System in Maywood, Illinois, Holly Kramer compared people with bigger belt sizes with thinner people: "We noted an approximate twofold increase in mortality risk once waist circumference exceeded 38.5 inches in females or greater than 44 inches in men."

STOP SMOKING, START LIVING LONGER

Tobacco is no doubt the single most cause of death in the world. Tobacco kills more than 5 million people which is much, much more than HIV/Aids, tuberculosis, malaria combined. By 2030 tobacco is going to kill 8 million people a year. If you smoke you are aging your lungs, heart, liver, digestive system, colon and sex organs at an astounding rate . . . your life expectancy is cut in half as is your nervous system functioning and brain cells.

Smoking, sugar intake, lack of exercise, loss of sleep, stress, loss of jobs and excess consumption have been the American habitat in pursuit of happiness, prosperity and fiscal stability . . . but like any "has been" the time for de-excessing is in order. Lower and healthier habit intake will provide better wellness outcomes. Experts have found diets that just lower consumption do not work for the long run . . . they reduce the short run consumption but fall victim to the habits that lurk in the subconscious. So the lasting changes in outcome must deal with the control of input consumption. "Read my mind" . . . it is mental and takes a reprogramming of the very reason for obesity and poor health . . . the need for a positive commitment to reform each individual's negative thinking not just their guilt triggers.

NATURAL BEAUTY STARTS WITH THE MIND AND ENDS WITH THE SIZE OF YOUR SELF-HEALTH SUCCESS. THE END ZONE IS ONLY A THOUGHT AWAY.

CHAPTER ELEVEN

What You Love and Hate Matters

- The most popular word in the human vocabulary is hate . . . I hate exercise . . . I hate being late . . . I hate my job . . . I hate the Cubs . . . I hate Mondays . . . etc.
- What do you love . . . that is what decides your health, happiness and prosperity.
- Love is the most used word in our dreams and hopes but not used to describe our lives . . . the Red Zone is bleak and hateful.
- The Self-Health Zone will require that you decide what you truly love and make it your thoughts, feelings then actions create a life fulfilled.

HUNTING RELATIONSHIPS

(Stop hunting for the better marriage by using this book to find the best in your current relationships, start renewing your feeling and power of love)

Are you ever happy with your situation or your job? If not how can you be happy with your wife, children, friends and self. Happiness should not come last . . . it has to come first for you to have good health and prosperity. You can be rich in dollars and poor in health and relationships.

Is this speculation or fact? Look at the statistics:

- Divorces over 50% of those who marry get divorced
- Drug use over 75% of those depressed actively use drugs, alcohol or substances to drop out
- Life expectancy

  o Females 80
  o Males 70

- Retirement

  o Females 62
  o Males 65

- Unemployment 9.3%
- Underemployment 16%-

Signs and symptoms of true youth:

- Happy
- Healthy
- Prosperous
- Faithful
- Positive
- Goal Seeking

What's your emotional, biological and mental age?

If you are emotionally old . . . the sun is setting on your future. No hope, no job, no marriage, no relationships, no life . . . If you are mentally old, the moon has eclipsed on your past, no dreams fulfilled, no love gained, no successful events, no joyful memories, no happy bed time stories, no value of life as you know it.

This state of affairs can and must be reversed for you to age naturally and happy and healthy, and prosperous. Many will just accept unhappiness as happenstance that one must endure, while in waiting for happenstance to change. Guess what, it does not happen if your stance is on blaming others or just good ole circumstance. Good luck on making that work.

The cure is, as always, in your head . . . you either think young or feel old . . . why not feel young and forget thinkin' old.

America is on the threshold of disaster economically, politically and emotionally due to the disintegration of the family unit. The dissolving of the most important of all relationships . . . marriage . . . be it same sex or not . . . we must reverse this trend or continue to be the rise and fall of America as was the Roman Empire, the Mayan Empire, the British Empire, etc.

Each individual in America must rethink their values using knowledge, study, thoughtful meditation and leadership . . . we can no longer leave this up to Government to dictate and police. Individual freedoms come from individual effort and we must go back to some basic values to repair what intellectual dominance has caused:

- Free to choose jobs
- Free to choose careers
- Free to choose leaders that value character
- Free to choose religious thought
- Free to take up arms only in our defense
- Free to represent peace rather than war
- Free to have housing, education and a standard of living that is experienced in varying degrees to all
- Free to pay taxes for the benefit of all
- Free to elect officials that are reachable and accountable to the voters.

Whether it be democrat or republican we need a more contrasting school of thought that takes us back to the founding fathers position that Government can be a blessing or a burden unless it is being reconstituted with new thought and representatives every 4 to 8 years . . . we have completely lost this with the advent of career politicians, state officials and their offspring dominating the power and funding to their benefit not the benefit of those that pay the majority of the bills, including their personal nest eggs . . . .

Einstein is famous for the theory of relativity as it applies to Science and it applies here: everything in humanity is relative to the acts of the majority and the minority shall not reject that for their own benefit.

Think about this before you think about yourself:

- 10% of the people lead the 90%
- 90% of the people would like to lead but don't
- Why not?

  o   Fear of the unknown
  o   Not goal driven
  o   Not prepared
  o   Not risk takers

- What does this have to do with aging?

  o   Fear causes stress that causes premature aging
  o   Goals are set but not pursued causing disappointment, stress and aging
  o   Little or no preparation causes failure, stress and aging
  o   Allowing ego to prevail causes selfishness, stress and aging
  o   Hiding behind excuses due to risk of rejection causes, hesitancy, stress and aging

Eliminate the above negatives and live for a stress free ageless life. Get involved and make a difference in your life, all Americans and the world.

Yes it is unique these days for baseball pitchers to win 20 games and marriages to last 50, 60, 70, 80 years . . . the world record seems to be 91 so we all have a ways to go.

My parents were married 50+ years, but due to poor health they expired in the 80's in nursing homes that were despicable to say the least. Shari's father died of cancer at the age of 66 much like Shari's sister. Can life style prevent cancer or other terminal diseases probably not directly but the way we think and act may create a different result. Only God knows the truth.

CHAPTER TWELVE

What You Pursue Matters

- Are goals real or just wishful thinking? Did we go to the moon? Did we build the skyscrapers? Did we beat polio? Are we ever going to have a peaceful world? The first 3 are goals while a peaceful world is an objective, not yet a goal to be attained.
- Objectives are plans but not commitments . . . goals are what we will decide to pursue.
- What are your Self-Health goals in your Red Zone world? Give it some thought and action and that pursuit will pay great dividends in your life.

START BELIEVING YOU ARE "NEVER TOO OLD TO LIVE"

Definition: old . . . past its time, out of stock, rickety, weak, no longer relevant, retired, over the hill, decrepit, out of touch, past its prime.

How many of us are willing to refer to ourselves as old? Probably 0% . . . if you believe you're old you are old at any age. My point we like to define old as someone else not us. Of course that is just a mental lapse since we probably don't exercise or eat right either.

Let's try another definition: old, little or no exercise, poor eating habits, stinkin' thinkin', hateful attitude, cynical, low esteem, unworthy, unemployed, divorced, sickly, dull, boring, unhappy, dead before death.

What's your emotional age versus your chronological age?

Dr.s Roizen and Oz have a web site where you can calculate your biological age compared to your chronological age . . . 360 some questions about your life style, ancestry, habits, goals, aspirations, relationships, etc. Most Americans are aging faster than their chronological age due to Red Zone life styles, habits and relationships. Of course the web site www.realage.com gives advice and exercises to move through the Red Zone to the Self-Health if you are willing to change your thinking, living habits and goals.

More importantly, what is your biological age versus your chronological age?

If you are 40 chronologically and 60 biologically you will die at least 20 years sooner than you should. On the other hand of you are 60 chronologically but 40 biologically life is under your control and you are in the Self-Health.

If you are emotionally old . . . the sun is setting on your future. No hope, no job, no marriage, no relationships, no life . . . If you are mentally old, the moon has eclipsed on your past, no dreams fulfilled, no love gained, no successful events, no joyful memories, no happy bed time stories, no value of life as you know it.

This state of affairs can and must be reversed for you to age naturally and happy and healthy, and prosperous. Many will just accept unhappiness as happenstance that one must endure, while in waiting for happenstance to change. Guess what, it does not happen if your stance is on blaming others or just good ole circumstance. Good luck on making that work.

The cure is, as always, in your head . . . you either think young or feel old . . . why not feel young and forget thinkin' old.

Rhonda Byrne in her timely and bestselling guide to happiness "The Secret", states: "life isn't happening to you, life is responding to you. Life is your call. You are the creator of your life. You decide what your life will be." You attract your own results through your own thoughts and actions.

Depok Chopra in his "7 Spiritual Laws of Success" establishes: that thinking, doing and finding happiness is a mental process from Karma(giving) to Dharma (finding your true talent and place in the Universe.

Dr. Venice Bloodworth in her book "The Key to Yourself" states: that an affirmation of "I am happy, healthy and prosperous" is not just words it is the retraining of the subconscious to be positive which is a principle of Universal law that puts aside the negative as being a result of not following Universal law.

Earle Nightengale in his teachings stated that "what you can conceive and believe you will achieve".

Eliminate the negatives and live for a stress free ageless life.

Being stress free is a process:

- Decide that you can overcome your fears . . . state them then confront them
- Set simple goals that can be accomplished then savor more ambitious successes
- Find a place for yourself satisfaction in giving to others and loving your present life
- Prepare each with a healthy agenda (age-nda means a health plan for the day including food, exercise, thoughts of love, acts of kindness)

- Stick your neck out for causes you stand for then take action to help others find their agenda
- What you reach is what you teach others. What you miss is what you are missing. Teach those you meet what they are missing.

The results are guaranteed:

1. You will be happier
2. You will be healthier
3. You will feel younger
4. You will not age due to stress

Sounds good but what can I do to get there? GET RID OF THE STRESS USING THIS SELF-HEALTH BOOK!

My wife's Aunt Edith was an example of laughter extending life's journey . . . she died at the age of 109 after being married 80 years to Uncle Ernie who was 101 when he moved on to the next continuum. Shari's mom Dorotha C. White was another of life's miracles . . . she was prematurely neglected and abuse in the nursing home system and expired at the age of 92, well on her way to 100 if circumstances had not intervened.

Compare her with her daughter Phyllis, Shari's sister who died of cancer at the age of 66 . . . irony never ceases in our Life stories. Shari and I are now in our seventies and convinced we can live to over 100 . . . our marriage of 54 years, 4 wonderful children and 12 gorgeous grandchildren and a brand new great grandson are hard to fathom but very heart warming.

Is this approach right for you . . . you need to answer that for your own self—satisfaction . . . we only know what works for us. But we do know that life is a gift that comes from the feeling of doing good, making a difference in others' lives virtually every way and every day . . . a life of feeling love for life itself. You are never too old to live this way.

An Ounce of Prevention is worth thousands of pounds of treatment . . . each of us have the best preventive system in the world our mind. Use it or lose it is also another profound bit of advice . . . have your mind use your immune system, your sub conscious system, your gut, you heart felt tendencies, your good habits are all a part of the functioning of that wonderful body you have. Health Science is now the driving force behind natural health movement to reduce Chronic disease without pills, chemicals, and traditional treatment using meditation, short burst of physical movements, walking, reading self-health books, separating the mind from the feelings to combat worry and fear which you yourself own until you discard them.

CHAPTER THIRTEEN

What You Avoid Matters (The Red Zone)

- Drugs are to be avoided.
- Alcohol, in excess and tobacco are the acceptable drugs that are just as destructive.
- Pornography, deviations and wrongful acts.
- Mental Commitment is not for everyone . . . the nonbelievers truly fall victim to their own reactions to circumstances.
- Just like the Bears, if you are ineffective in moving past the goal line out of the RED ZONE you will lose every battle and the war against bad habits.

SELF-HEALTH PRACTICED

You are the only one that can determine your life time . . . if you can outrun the driver of the car you are one of the more fit . . . so the definition of Self-Health was the most important information you can receive:

S cience
E ngineered
L ife
F ulfillment

H ow you are thinking determines your weight
E ating when you are hungry and stopping when you are full
A ging is not a factor in measuring your longevity
L ife is now your show and stage so act on it
T ime is now an ally in your use of it
H ealth is your journey not a destination

Healthy . . . Body . . . Mind . . . Heart . . .
Soul = is your Self Health

Why would the avoidance of chemicals and certain behaviors defer aging?

Drugs are to be avoided . . . then why do so many people use them? It is the Red Zone subconscious mind that creates fears and depression triggers that lead to poor health, unhappiness and poverty. Is it the lack of will to resist that brings us down or is it the need to find the courage to confront our fears? The experts contend that the use of chemicals is much less worse than the pain of depression and fear. Finding a faith in pursuing a Self-Health life style usually takes a negative outcome to create the reason to suffer through the depression to the joy of accomplishment . . . which I have found in exercise . . . physical or mental.

Alcohol, in excess and tobacco are the acceptable drugs that are just as destructive to the Self-Health life style. Society has its own mechanisms for judging and inciting the use of other habitual stimulants that inhibit the pursuit of happiness, health and prosperity. It becomes incumbent on the mind of the user to find the reason for quitting is stronger than the bad behavior that it causes.

Pornography, deviations and wrongful acts are Red Zone activities to be avoided if your focus is on health, happiness and prosperity. Deviation is very personal and erosion to self-health and its benefits. We all have our moments of desire and fantasizing something more exciting than we have . . . but in the long run this is just another distraction from having control of the short run impulses that will prevent aging according to natural events rather than unnatural desires.

The commitment to Self-Health habits is not for everyone . . . the non-believers truly fall victim to their own reactions to circumstances not realizing that the cure is in their head waiting to be activated. This is called the universal law of attraction. Once activated the creative mind can take you there as the law of nature that controls all our spirits. Whether you deem it God or the Universal Mind it certainly makes the journey more enjoyable and meaningful.

Just like the Super Bowl winner, that is the most effective moving into the END ZONE you will win every battle and the war against bad habits. This impacts your health, wealth, happiness and relationships. In a life of 65 years it may be your choice to live it up and disregard the physical and mental warnings until it is too late . . . or you may hit your limit or bottom or loss so it is no longer acceptable to be a reactionary but a visionary for your own longevity.

Avoidance is the same as faith . . . when you believe in your own choices for the sake of others and you feel good about being fit your mind is connected to the Universal Mind . . . that is taking us to the embraces of love and happiness.

Chapter Fourteen

What You Feel You're Worth Matters

- Would you wager your life on a lottery ticket or Russian Roulette? Is that all you are worth? Each individual values themselves every day by their actions. The Red Zone thinkers are the malcontents, street people, criminal minds and destructive forces in the world.
- Those actions create results that are directed by feelings coming from each subconscious mind . . . if you have low self-esteem or worth you lower yourself to that level . . . it is correctable in your Self-Health program.
- As a society we must correct this type of thinking because it is how we will be thinking of ourselves when we cannot afford the health care costs to treat such behaviors.
- Realistically, this is the responsibility of every American to work on their self-capital and how it contributes to the Greater Good and invested in the American Enterprise.

Would you wager your life for money . . . for a new job . . . a new wife . . . a better home; probably not. It doesn't make sense that you wager your life on a life style dictated by a subconscious out of control. Controlling the mind is an exercise in good judgment and understanding of self—confidence that you are doing the right thing . . . Self-Health thinking is what we need. But it is gained with some pain. Personal affirmations repeated and repeated until they become beliefs in the subconscious. Actions create results that are directed by feelings coming from each subconscious mind . . . if you have low self-esteem or worth you lower yourself to that level . . . it is correctable in your Self-Health program.

Beyond sounding preachy changing habits is the technique for making the transformation from the Red Zone to the Self-Health in your own space. The researchers were looking for a silver bullet for the masses and are finding that it is a personal commitment to change life styles and that usually means a sacrifice in the mind of the beholder who may not be there yet. Like any other addiction poor habits are acquired not inherited so the change must be done mentally prior to making the changes physically.

Some will do this at a young age because of inheriting a life style from their parents be that good or bad, most times picking up on their bad habits as much if not more than their good habits. The definition of habits is something that is done without thinking and precautions on a routine basis. My habits are not inherited due to a rejection of the life style my parents exhibited. They did me a favor by not embracing me in an sort of way and allowed me to develop my own dreams, schemes and foibles. My children on the other hand have been greatly influenced by my wife's and my habits and aspirations . . . most are good. Is this bragging . . . I guess it is but that is what this book is about . . . my and my wife's good luck when it comes to health, happiness and prosperity. But, like any opportunity it has been hard earned and appreciated by our results . . . four grown children who are well adjusted, twelve grandchildren who are well adjusted and a new great grandson who looks to be, because of his parents on his way to health, happiness and prosperity.

On the other hand I don't discount my parents influence . . . my father never had any liquor in our home, never swore, worked for the same factory for 33 years and was honest as the day was long. He was a staunch union supporter. His family was farmers in Iowa and worked until they died (most in their 70' or 80's). My mother came from a dysfunctional home with a tragic impact on her. However, she like my father worked very hard, provided my sister and I with homemade clothes, the latest in shoes, music and dance lessons. She never swore, drank but did steal away with her cigarettes. Both only had an eighth grade education and never felt equal to their kids who got college educations, good jobs and career paths out of our home town of Indianola Iowa.

Without this upbringing, though done without expressions of love, provided the security and freedom for my sister and I to make our own way without baggage which is very important to being able to do it your own way.

Is this the solution for most Americans . . . no. Most have way more baggage than I had and my wife is a great influence on my life and our children. She is a farm girl until seventh grade with a very happy home life and great self-image. You can tell that in her picture in Chapter Ten.

In football I learned that the quarterback was the boss . . . in baseball it was the shortstop and in basketball it was the point guard . . . those were the positions that I chose for my self-worth. The problem was I was too small for being the starter in any of these sports. I was the sixth man in basketball, the second string quarterback and did not start in any sport except baseball in my senior year. But this was setting me up for a life of taking risks in business and in life. I started my own business at the age of 37 and a new line of business at the age of 70 . . . always feeling like I can succeed if I work hard.

Well working hard is not enough . . . it takes faith, control over my emotions, feelings for other people, patience, overcoming fear, defeat, disappointment and distraction. All in a day's work for an enterprise that has all the obstacles as well . . . nursing homes. I decide long ago to pursue a specialty in health care where no one else had established a solution for aging and dying. Now that I have held myself out to be a health care guru more obstacles crop up . . . regulators, bankers, tax accountants and experts everywhere telling me I am wrong at the right time and right at the wrong time. Still I persist with my writings and doings.

Why not . . . my wife, son and I are proving that nursing homes can be respectable but not homes to the patients . . . we are an alternative to their own home. We focus on getting them back to independence or some semblance of that so they can be self-supporting as much as possible. The setting is academic . . . it is the actual feeling of self-worth that we work with so the person can have a quality of life in those years before the next stepping stone.

American Enterprise has given me and my family good health, happiness and prosperity and not without risk. My first business venture was an accounting firm, consulting practice and a computer software company specializing in nursing homes. I spread myself and my resources too thin and ended up in Chapter 11 bankruptcy seeking the court's protection. I started over and paid back my debtors but it took 18 years during which time I could not own a home and was treated like dirt by the IRS until I paid my debt to society. But we never faltered in our faith that we were going to someday make a difference in the nursing home business.

For the next twenty years my wife, son and I traveled to twenty-two states with our software and consulting services assisting 145 nursing homes in improving their Medicare business and profitability. Our true mission was to acquire enough capital to buy our own facilities because we still did not feel the industry was headed in the right direction. So in September 2009 we acquired our first nursing home and since then two more. We thought we knew the business until we ran head on to the regulators. It is not the regulations that are inhibiting it is the misinterpretation, arbitrary and capricious way the Government treats nursing homes. Due to poor care in the past and the application of minimum standards and antiquated payment methods by the Federal and State Government officials, the nursing homes are the whipping post of health care.

Our business plan was to acquire small town nursing homes, restore them and set up a franchise business so local businessmen and women could run them. Take corporate America out of pyramiding them into poor care and bad press. Well that ended when were hit by Gestapo tactics by the State of Iowa and almost put out of business before we got started. (Go to Appendix I and II for the gory details of AMERICA IN THE RED ZONE).

Chapter Fifteen

What You Give Matters

- "You get in proportion to what you give" . . . sound familiar? All philosophers and psychologists pound away at this one. But the Red Zone thinkers say "do unto others before they do it to you".
- Who is right? The Self-Health program stresses that fear and stress are our biggest enemies, not other human beings. So why fight each other when we can give ourselves to others so they can in return give to us?
- However, the giver must act first then the rewards of receiving comes to us ten—fold in better health, happiness and abundance. It is universal law taught by the greatest leaders of all time. Be one yourself.

EXERCISE GIVING

(Stop hunting for a better job by using this book to exercise giving to your current job, start working for others' dreams)

My wife is the most giving person I have known . . . as a result everyone around her respects her opinion and her actions because she is we centered not me centered.

I have to work every day at being as good as she is . . . her first thought is of the other person. My first thought tends to be about my wishes, dreams and goals. Together we have built a wonderful life of having it out every six months because I step out of the acceptable bounds of what is reasonable and likely to happen . . . the dreamer brought down to earth. She the GOOD WILL FINDER stating the obvious to consider best decisions for all involved not just my limited perception and far out vision.

To be a good giver you must exercise the will to be good not just a "emotion giver". The emotion giver gives for personal reasons such as a disaster needing contributions, a tip for a table, a shallow commitment for volunteerism, small gifts to the pan handler, etc.

The traits of my wife the GOOD GIVER:

- Doesn't consider the amount as being a factor
- Responds to need not who is needy
- Follows through on volunteer work
- Doesn't say no to the kids, grandkids or in laws
- Brings a present whenever she feels like giving, which is on all occasions, including vacation shopping for trinkets
- Always says yes to requests for the check

As a result she is ageless, she is beauty, she is the smile that lights up the room, she is the center of our family's root system and my wings. God has blessed us with her, her mother and her mother's mother who were all givers.

I am still learning the act of giving . . . not just advice as I am attempting to do in this book . . . but actually being better at being a human being:

1. Look past self for my worth
2. Take time to volunteer
3. Take time to get involved in Governing

4. Take time to make a difference in the life of aging America
5. Be active in bringing America back to a giving country standing for peace rather than a threatening force using imperialism . . . which means less military and more charity to those that need liberty but don't want it

G ifts
I mprove
V irtually
E verything

Sam Walton in his book "Made in America" stated that his only regret was not discovering the power of sharing his wealth with his employees (associates) earlier. America's wealthy give more away than they keep.

CHAPTER SIXTEEN

What You Believe In Matters

- Are your answers in the Bible? Or are they coming from your own head before you can stop and think. I call this Red Zone thinking.
- Belief and faith are big things when it comes to health, happiness and prosperity.
- What you conceive, believe you can achieve according to the great thinkers in the Self-Health End Zone.
- For simple results we all must rethink how we respond to each decision we make because it determines our life's outcome . . . so believe you can achieve the Self-Health principles and run with it.

All Americans have the right to stay healthy, for the greater good.

My mother and father were old when they were in their forties, characterized by their use of false teeth, thoughts of early retirement, being out of shape, being in poor health, and destined to be in a nursing home living out their final years in miserable conditions. They were both victims of eldercide or the systematic institutionalization of the elderly after a chronic illness.

I, at the age of seventy-four, on the other hand, have all my teeth; think in terms of late retirement; am in the best shape I can be in; am taking no medications; have less than 10% body fat; am a cross-trainer, tennis player, photographer, and author; and am destined to avoid institutional confinement for as long as humanly possible. Having my own business with my wife and son as partners is the motivation for my most productive life beginning at seventy, together with my three daughters who all are career businesswomen and looking forward to late retirement.

My wife, also has all her teeth, beautiful hair, enviable figure, and a no Botox face who wants to stay in business with me for the duration; has a pace maker for a congenital heart condition; does yoga, tennis, and treadmill; and will be with me in business and as my life partner until the time we cast our last line in the ocean of opportunity.

For us our most productive life truly has begun with our commitment to a life style of love and family. However, looking around at our peers, the future is not so bright; most people our age opted for early retirement, do little if any exercise, have bad food choices, accept being overweight, are out of work, and are unhappy. To us this is not the American dream. It is going to be a nightmare for our economy, our health care system, and our children who will have to suffer with us in our old age and a society that thinks living unhappily past sixty-five is all we can expect. I have nothing but hope for our situation and nothing but fear for the majority of aging Americans that are going to expect to be housed, fed, diaper changed, and pushed around in a wheelchair. If that is the American Dream then let me on the next spaceship to Mars.

If this sounds self-serving, it is. Our political system, economics, and work life are predicated on each of us pursuing happiness in a free and democratic society so we can retire early with no financial obligations, and not being institutionalized because we failed to prepare for aging. But our politicians, big government, and employers do not act in the best interests of the big picture. Spend now, worry later; tax less, borrow more; and use credit to fund the high life now, apply for Medicaid later. Tax the folks, milk the goats for income not outcome.

What we should do is make due like life begins at seventy (give me an economic incentive to accomplish the moral incentives of living longer and better):

LR = Late retirement incentives—those who work beyond seventy years old will pay no taxes and will receive free health care if they have a job.

LGGL = Lose you gain and gain you lose tax credits—those who lose weight to their ideal body weight get a 15% tax credit and those who gain beyond their ideal body weight pay an additional 15% tax surcharge.

FC = First-class seats on airlines at 70% off the airfare.

FP = Free pass to membership in the American Association of Late Retirees (AALR).

Since the AARP has turned into an insurance company and a lobbyist, those who are members can be better served with a practical avoidance of over medication, re-hospitalization, and chronic diseases, none of which AARP has a clue about preventing. The baby boomers need health preservation, not pay more and more for illness; wellness is cheaper and much more enjoyable.

As for the health care professionals, it might behoove them to join the AALR movement so they can be a part of the culture to keep Americans healthy so we all can be wealthy in life after seventy, rather than dead by seventy by fat ingestion.

Jerry Rhoads

For me mental and physical exercise has enabled me to overcome a negative self-image, a fear of the unknown, because I now can control my thoughts about what I want and it will appear as it has for many others who believe they can, have the will and it becomes what they are.

110

CHAPTER SEVENTEEN

What You Will Stand Up For Matters

- A great quote is "if you stand for nothing, you will fall for anything"! What do you really stand for . . . better health, being happy for a change and gaining wealth, instead of weight, as a result of feeling good about what you do?
- That is the Self-Health . . . this does not require money, cheating or pain . . . it is not too hard to attain or make gains . . . it is a commitment to a change in life style that uses the following 10 commandments for America to ultimately exit the "Red Zone" into the Self-Health End Zone, as a country.

TEN COMMANDMENTS MOVING FROM THE RED ZONE TO THE SELF-HEALTH

1. Self-Health programs for preventing chronic illnesses, obesity and depression.
2. Reduction of chemicals ingested by Americans.
3. Physical and mental exercising that fights off obesity and depression.
4. Health preservation initiatives by health and fitness experts.
5. De-institutionalization of the elderly and disabled.
6. Natural health remedies promoted and provided by health professionals.

7. Most importantly resources used to pay for outcomes not incomes . . . define outcomes as the reduction of known health and illness problems . . . not just symptomatic guesses or medical diagnosis without root cause analysis.
8. Replace inductive pursuit of treatment to deductive pursuit of cause and effect.
9. Get Government out of the health care business and eliminate 60% of the wasted resources.
10. Elect government officials that have knowledge and expertise in Health Care delivery and funding.

PHYSICAL EXERCISING AFFECTS THE OTHER NINE—GETTING IN THINKING SHAPE LEADS YOU TO PHYSICAL WELL BEING

(Stop being a couch potato by using this book to do physical exercises, start being an action hero) USE THE DOWNSIZER SPREAD SHEET to plan your Body Mass Index—a target for self-health . . . available online at www.nevertoooldtolive.com

Preaching won't work when it comes to getting you to exercise . . . typically Americans do not, will not and cannot exercise. Why? Because we do not see the importance of feeling pain . . . because exercise does require some pain. Be it loss of breath, soreness of muscle mass, mental aversion, not enough time, too little results instantly.

I for one have exercised all my life . . . I do not consciously know why . . . I hate the thought of it every day . . . but I do it. Why? I guess it is a habit formed in my formative years and it has stuck in my subconscious forcing me to feel guilty if I don't do it.

How can you form a feeling of guilt by avoiding the very thing that will allow you to live healthier, longer and in some energy form forever? Thoughts create action . . . think about getting it over with but feel good after it is. Yes it has to be a habit formed from your desire to live for longer. If you do not work on this thought process you will not even live as long as you should. You will die with the following profile:

- At least 50 pounds over your ideal body weight
- At least 4 to 5 chronic diseases
- At least 10 medications per day
- At least some days in a wheel chair
- At least some days in a diaper
- At least 5 years in a nursing home
- At least 10 times per year in the emergency room
- At least 5 times per year admitted to the hospital
- At least 15 times per year to the doctor

This is the fate of at least 65% of Americans and is increasing at an unbelievable rate. Not only does this impact your life it impacts all of our lives . . . the cost of unhealthy Americans is over $3 trillion per year along with the stress of premature dying rather than healthful living.

Just as in mental exercising we must make a personal commitment to change our thinking because that is what changes our daily behavior.

What could the daily behavior be?

1. Walk instead of ride . . . cars, bikes, stairs, jogs, roller skates, roller blades, ice skates

   a. Walking 30 minutes per day burns 300 calories that you would not have burned . . .
   b. that amounts to over 10,000 calories per year or a loss of twenty pounds . . .
   c. in six short months the average American could be at 85% of their best body mass . . .

2. Working in the yard burns 350 calories per hour,
3. Working on or cleaning your own car burns 200 calories per hour
4. Using Wii for exercise games rather than violent games (burns 100's of calories with continued use)
5. Participating in sports (tennis burns 400 calories in an hour, softball burns 300 calories per 7 innings, running burns 400 calories in 30 minutes, bowling burns 200 calories per 10 frames, golf carrying your bag for 18 holes burns 500 calories)
6. Even chewing gum supposedly burns 100 calories an hour . . . that isn't even painful

What are the odds that you will take this seriously?

- There are 1.7 million patients in nursing homes
- There are 3 million residents in assisted living facilities
- There are 8 billion prescription drugs used annually in nursing homes
- There are 5 million admissions annually to hospitals
- There are 6 million ER visits to hospitals per year
- There are 77 million fairly unhealthy baby boomers that retire this decade
- There are 550,000 premature deaths in nursing homes every year

What if you do not take this seriously?

- America's health care costs exceed $2 trillion per year
- Life expectancy for the first time ever is going down
- Life expectancy for parents are higher than their children's will be
- More and more of our children will not outlive their parents

Make your choice now or you will never make it . . . if you walk by a crack in the sidewalk once you will never see it again. If you decide to be healthy you will be . . . your mind will take your body there.

Jerry Rhoads in his book Eldercide points out that aging Americans are being institutionalize against their will when the families can no longer take care of their decline. To remedy Eldercide and Restore Elderpride takes the prevention pill as well as the prescription pill. Annually 550,000 human beings die in nursing homes . . . many if most prematurely and costly to the health and welfare of America. It is our responsibility we preserve our health not destroy it and suffer the consequences . . . . otherwise Eldercide and its devastating losses face us all.

SELF-HEALTH ACHIEVED

You are now the one that determines your life time, weight, happiness, longevity . . . unless you can out run the car you will never be passive again . . . so the achievement of Self-Health ends with you:

S cience
E ngineered
L ife
F ulfillment

H ow you think and act determines your weight
E at only when you are hungry and always stop when you are full
A ging is a biological formula to measure your true longevity
L ife is your show and stage so act as if you will die tomorrow
T ime is a chronological factor only if you misuse it
H ealth is your journey not a dreaded destination

CHAPTER EIGHTEEN

The Self-Health End Zone

— Thinking END ZONE diet is about changing your self-worth
— Acting diet as if you already have the self-worth
— Eating diet for your-self-worth not your anxieties
— Loving diet with those that are helping you change
— Giving diet to reward those that are supporting your change
— Believing diet to attain your desired self-image
— Working diet attaining your goals not setting unattainable limits
— Health diet is your responsibility to American society
— Wealth diet is your reward for thinking well of yourself
— Prosperity diet is happiness for all in the SE LF-HEALTH end zone

Have you ever thought about the weight, height, look, attitude and pride you would like to live with? All of these are at your disposal except height . . . that is the only one that you are stuck with, like it or not. According to the experts on life style you are what you think you are . . . so a thinking diet would help take you out of the Red Zone into the Self-Health. The only limitation is your approach to what life throws your way. Obstacles, disappointments, failures, broken promises, hurt feelings are always going to come your way but you need to respond to those in a hopeful and positive manner . . . this is where the Thinking Diet comes into play. Diet yourself to positive responses to negative events, thoughts and circumstances and your life is guaranteed to be what you want it to be.

This is called the Acting Diet . . . making believe you already have what you want . . . life styles are made not inherited. Self-worth or lack thereof is dictating your mood, your habits, your results unless you capture your subconscious and mold it into what you can do not what you can't do. Personal affirmations verbalized to oneself will reprogram how you feel about yourself so you feel good about what you are thinking and Acting positively will follow.

The Loving Diet is touted to be the potion for embracing life for another so we can connect and procreate. To practice the loving diet should be the easiest of the diets . . . but for many it is the most elusive. It takes two to love and we mammals seem hung up on formalities like sexual orientation, personal frailties, greed, selfishness, pride, anger, temperament, to a fault. Overcoming this self-centered world we are born into takes relaxing our need to be dominant and become a partner in life with someone you feel passionate about. For love is the most positive act in our daily living and our longevity . . . it is not only a stressful event in its gestation but it is a stress reliever in its role in pursuing dreams and counting blessings.

Give and you shall receive is a diet of intentions . . . do we really need to give without strings attached. Only heart strings for another person or persons demonstrates a sincere gift. So the Giving Diet is more than material items . . . it is immaterial thoughts that are converted to material actions . . . money given because giving is immaterial to wealth but material to the needy. When the Red Cross solicits help for hurricane Sandy and we respond it is for material purposes but immaterial to our true since of giving because the recipient is too far removed to become our responsibility. Giving time to the Red Cross on the other hand is personal and more of a Gift than money. Giving to our children love and boundaries for behavior are the greatest gifts of all . . . it either starts the cycle or continues the cycle we learned from our parents. A Diet of Giving rhymes with living that is achieving that rhymes with receiving a life of happiness.

What you believe in commits you to some form of action . . . be it right wrong or indifferent you are in motion. The Believing Diet recommends that this be done with fore thought and an expectation that it has already happened and all you need to do is counts your achievements. Some call this dreams and schemes but in the real world of self-attainment and the Law of Attraction the mind that conceives, and believes achieves before it becomes a conscious reality . . . it is planting the seed and expecting it to grow into a beautiful crop of abundant successes as one who receives in proportion to what one believes.

Work is a four letter word avoided by many and cherished by the rest of us. Without it we are victims and with it we are heroes. The Working Diet is not drudgery or painful if done for one's self esteem . . . pursue your dreams and be happy with the work it takes to achieve them. However, it must be meaningful work and joyful in its effort and productive in its results. So the mind creating the work and the products of their labor are the backbone of Capitalism and Enterprise . . . invest the capital so a creative mind can conceive a saleable product that produces a profit to restore the consumed capital. The cycle represents our economy, our education system, our political system, our foreign policy, our social system our fulfillment of human capital.

Health is a form of wealth if based on wellness not illness . . . pursuing treatment of illnesses has been the foundation of our physician and hospital practices with the other providers following suit. Now that illness is procreating other illnesses we must stop and reconsider that Health is a Diet of prevention and preservation habits that do not require pills and multiple ER visits to produce quality of life. It requires self-health practiced by all Americans to be able to prevent chronic illnesses and preserve a healthy life style. It takes mental exercising as much as physical exercising because the mind is the director and the body is the employer of better habits to overcome the subconscious habits we have inherited from our parents and the conventional American culture.

The definition of Wealth diet is more than money less than mind over matter but making healthy decisions matter. For the wealth we all seek in the aging process is to be able to live happily, healthy and prosperous. To get there starts with our thinking, then our feeling, then with our doing. None of us are born with this process ingrained in our minds . . . just the opposite. Our parents and society have told us consistently what not to do not what to do . . . so we do what the conditioning has done, so we do what we were told not to do because our subconscious mind does to discern the difference. It only knows action not what is good for us and what is bad. That has to be a conscious effort to change our subconscious responses. If that makes sense then you are on your way to changing your subconscious into a conscious field of dreams.

Prosperity is the culmination of the preceding diets of heart, mind, muscle and soul . . . you are never too old to live right and to change bad habits into a fulfilling life style that allows you to age naturally and stress free.

STRESS FREE AGING

(Stop cynical complaining about politics, religion, sex, taxes, money and social obstacles to your success . . . by using this book you can find your role and acceptance of these situations and put them in perspective for your stress free life . . . start being a part of the solutions).

Jerry Rhoads

I catch myself these days complaining about everything that seems outside of my circle of influence . . . maybe I am assuming I am perfect and no one else is . . . what a flawed approach to life. I am working on being more receptive to what appears to be stupid and is really another view point that I do not agree with.

If I accomplish this learning curve I will have much less stress in my life and more receptive listeners to my life style opinions.

Yes there is much to complain about . . . negative influences put you in a negative frame of mind if you let it . . . I am stopping that as of now. And so can you . . . think better live longer, happier, healthier more prosperous lives.

Stress . . . the act of letting things get to you. De-Stressers . . . the act of avoiding or counteracting things that get to you.

- Aches and pains . . . exercise until you avoid them
- Worries and concerns . . . counteract them with thoughts of joy, happiness and hope
- Financial and economic threats . . . think about solutions not the problems . . . creative thinking is spurred by exercise more than any other act
- Personal tragedies and emotional depression . . . get the mind and body working for a common cause either in exercise or in work related activities
- Getting old before your time . . . if you have abused your mind and body for years a reversal will take some stress relievers every day . . . better activities of daily living (diet, exercise, meditation and hopefulness) . . . if you are not able to do this you have given in the inevitable health and aging issues . . . stop them now and forever be grateful that you did.

The results are guaranteed:

- You will be happier
- You will be healthier
- You will feel younger
- You will not age due to stress

The beneficiaries will be:

- Family
- Business associates
- Relatives
- Friends
- Yourself

The transition from the Red Zone to the End Zone revolves around the three "C's" . . . commitment to self-health, creation of your dream machine (your subconscious mind) and climaxing with of a life of aging naturally that until now seemed elusive to your desires. Believe it and it will come unto you.

EPILOGUE

Aging in Place—Can We Afford It?
(taken from the Jerry Rhoads' book
"The Boomers Are Coming")

The academics have come up with another catch all solution for the Baby Boomers hitting 60—Aging in Place—where everyone basks in the safety of their own home until they die from natural causes with relatives looking in on them. In fact, "Aging in Place" according to the academics, means that the culture of the past is now the home of the future. The use of terms like primary care, medical homes, bundled payment, managed populations, community based services, block grants for Medicaid, end of life care, fraud and abuse, enforcement, ACO's, CCP's, are the Government's attempt to control the money not the quality.

Of course this cannot and will not happen due to the extreme cost of having the providers travel from home to home providing treatment then transporting the patients to hospitals for average lengths of stay of 2 days for tests and surgery. Then back home to recover and be functional without a support system. The other obstacle to this approach is the lack of scientific definition of what causes chronic diseases and how we can prevent illness and pursue wellness for the benefit of aging America. Health care delivery is the venue of managing the aging process better using wellness habits not managing mass population's cultural habits.

If Aging in Place and health preservation for preventing diseases are to have a chance at ever working, many changes must take place in the home and in our society:

- Fitness and nutrition must be put in place and adhered to.
- Chronic disease needs to be prevented.
- Work life cannot end at 65.
- The home must be set up to accept some disabilities.
- Transportation for the disabled must be designed for ease of use.
- Health care insurance must pay for preventing disease and preserving health.
- The government needs to standardize what they are going to pay for and honor the commitment, regardless of the economics.
- Wasted resources must be removed from health care practices using technology, payment incentives and care planning.
- Politicians should not have the final call on allocation of resources.
- Performance must be the basis for payment, supported by evidence of what the payment is pursuing and attainment of a positive outcome.

The idea that Aging in Place means every home must be a nursing home, an emergency room, a doctor's office and a place to die is not a feasible or rational solution. Here's why:

Fitness and Nutrition

The lack of these two intangibles, which causes almost all tangible chronic diseases, are the bane of the health care system in America. Very few Baby Boomers have a commitment to staying fit and avoiding weight problems. However, without some change in the cultural mores for these vital ingredients, the concept of Aging in Place is just another facade. Only 15% of Americans over 65 exercise on a regular basis and 75% are overweight. We are told that most of our problems are genetic . . . the aging gene . . . the personality gene . . . the social gene . . . the fat gene . . . are to blame for our maladies. As long as we believe this, the more we will believe that the answer is in a pill. We are not aging in place, we are dying in place.

Solution: America's health is dependent on fitness and nutrition. For our society to function in a worldwide competitive market, we must create economic incentives for our citizens to pursue and preserve health. The use of tax deductions for fitness and nutrition expenses is a must. Higher premiums for the unhealthy who pay their own costs are the only way to bring resources in balance with the demand. By taking the employer out of the equation, we put the onus of health care costs on the offenders.

Prevention of chronic disease

45% of the health care dollar is spent on the five most prevalent chronic diseases (diabetes, obesity, cardiovascular disease, hypertension, and lung disease). No discernible work has been done by the FDA on pharmaceuticals as the perpetrator of medications causing as many chronic diseases as they presume to fix. By destroying the ability of the immune system to ward off common ailments, we are being set up for the dependence on and destruction of the human genome. Looking at the other side of the coin, reduction of prescription drugs and increases in natural remedies allow the body to adapt to the viruses and bacteria that have been around since the beginning of time.

Granted, the life expectancy rose to all time heights until obesity entered the scene. We give credit to the American health care system for the improvement, however, most deaths are attributable to smoking, drinking, criminal acts, wars, sexual transmitted problems, suicide, murder, neglect and abuse. Not until we began treating every malady with a pill did we increase the incidence of conditions like diabetes, vascular constriction, hypertension, cancer, respiratory problems, weight gain, dementia, autism, and birth defects.

Solution: Not every health problem lends itself to medication. Physicians need to become better educated on how to avoid prescriptions, rather than use them as a guesstimate on treating symptoms. The answer includes mandating care plans, eliminating phone orders for drugs, and interacting with elderly patients for their physical, emotional and social restorative functioning.

Work life ending at 65

What a concept when, in the past, most people died at the age of 45. The faulty thinking is that if we can live until 65, we should never have to work again. Now that life expectancy is 78, why are we still counting on 65 as the age of retirement? Looking at the new levels for life expectancy, we should be retiring at 98, not 65.

We have trapped our society with empty nesters who are not gainfully occupied, sitting around getting obese, and dependent on prescription drugs. Of course, economically, we cannot afford for anyone to retire unless they are wealthy because our society has left everything to the politicians to decide.

The corporate giants, the Federal Government, and the health care professionals all tell us when to retire and have promised the full payment plan through pensions and Social Security. Unfortunately, they miscalculated by a few trillion. According to statistics, the Federal Government is $100 trillion in the hole right now, using generally accepted accounting principles, and the numbers are getting worse each day. Our Senators and Representatives have their health care benefits and retirement plans, thanks to the taxpayer. It is the ordinary taxpayer that does not have a nest egg. They are too busy trying to pay taxes and stay afloat.

Solution: Retirement is not the end all. For a society that is built on productive activities, it makes no sense for people who live to be 90 to be out of the work environment for 25 years. There are plenty of jobs for older Americans if we focus on forming a health preservation culture of more spas, more gyms, more health clubs, more testing, screening and preventive interventions. There are plenty of jobs that can be created by replacing the institutional bias for treatment with proactive plans for health preservation.

The Home Set-up

99% of homes today are not conducive to handling disabilities, let alone an aging in place society. Aging in Place proposes that all medical services are delivered to the person's home. That means for the low functioning elderly, someone has to be in the home 24 hours per day for the activities of daily living (ADL's = eating, bathing, dressing, grooming, toileting, walking). This does not come cheap. Also, there can be no stairs in the way of a wheelchair or a walker, carpeting that causes falls, chemicals within reach due to dementia and not knowing what not to drink, or access to stoves or heat controls, due to loss of memory and reasoning.

Solution: The high functioning can be at home to a degree, however, when the ADL's deteriorate, congregate living is the only solution. With this scenario, we still have the problem of fixing meals, going to the store, driving to the doctor and climbing stairs. Some states theorize that they can employ relatives to be at home caregivers. However, what about training for the caregivers? What about the statistic that 80% of the financial and physical abuse toward the elderly in the home is perpetrated by a relative? In effect, if the assisted living and nursing homes were organized around the concept of restoring the elderly so they could live more independently, then Aging in Place might have a future. Right now, we have dying in place.

Transportation adapted to disabilities of aging

Visual and cognitive impairment are the two most prevalent maladies for the aging population, causing 75% of the accidents for drivers over 65. Since our most accessible mode of transportation is the automobile, adapting the automobile for these physical impairments is not an option. The answer needs to be public transportation, and it must be accessible to wheelchairs, walkers and for low strength usage. In effect, the biggest obstacle for Aging in Place is lack of transportation. In emergencies, we have ambulances. In scheduled situations, we have a neighbor or relative. For mobility, we have nothing. The typical 80 year old should not be driving in traffic and has limited reaction to what is destined to happen . . . a red light . . . a stop sign . . . a child running across a street . . . a snow storm . . . a rain storm.

Solution: We have congregate living for a reason. We can provide better services using economies of scale, rather than duplicating what can be provided en masse. Again, the current service industry for the elderly must change its infrastructure, not society. It is much quicker for the local nursing home to be required to provide restorative care before they get paid than to devise a more costly method that has no prospects of meeting the demands of the Baby Boomers. All of the discussions should be about modifying the current service mechanism, rather than devising an unattainable goal.

Getting Old Insurance

Our current health care system was designed to treat, not prevent or restore. So, the proposal for physicians and hospitals to be in the business of preventing the very thing that puts money in their pockets seems ludicrous to them. However, if we don't change the paradigm, no one will have a job without paying for health care for themselves and for other people. 80% of the current health care dollar is spent in the last two years of people's lives. And, these lives are not admirable. If we only had a concept where we all, from cradle to grave, financed our own health and welfare programs. Then, as we decide to stay healthy, we could save our own money, not our employer's or the Government's money.

Solution: The current talk is about universal health care at no cost to the individual. Letting someone else pay for your poor health decisions is, of course, flawed logic. The cost control that we seek is unattainable because the only person that can exert that control is not paying the bill. How can we totally revamp a system that has been in place for 50 years? Either go broke, then do it because we have to, or be proactive and make a comprehensive change, so we can have the following:

- Standardized benefits for all Americans (ISO 9000 standards).
- Mandated processes that require standardized terminology for computerizing and economizing the cost.
- Meaningful database for diagnostics, evidenced based modeling of the care plan, and execution of care supported by outcome based documentation.
- Use of the problems and programs in the care plan to determine pay for results.
- Payment of outcomes to measure the quality of life in our congregate living, assisted living, nursing homes and home care.
- Care plans for costing the care, billing the outcomes and eliminating wasted resources in facilities (turnover, absenteeism, injury, theft, abuse, neglect, inefficiency, low productivity and poor quality).

he bottom line is to save $400 to $600 billion per year in waste, with better quality of life for an aging America.

Government commitment

A universal health care program cannot be administered by the Federal and State Governments. Whether it is $2 trillion or $4 trillion, it will never be enough. The Bureaucracy and 39,000 pages of regulations supporting the taxing and health care systems let the criminals hide and steal.

Most people and providers are well meaning, however, the current enforcement mentality alleges that everyone is suspect and guilty until proven innocent. This has not worked for the IRS and does not work for CMS (Centers for Medicare & Medicaid Services). Any funding for universal coverage must be administered by private businesses, dedicated to saving money from eliminating waste, and excelling in the prevention of chronic disease and preservation of the health of an aging society.

Solution: The infrastructure exists for the collection and distribution of the American Health Insurance Program. Current HMO's, PPO's, managed care organizations, disease management companies, and health care insurance underwriters all have a vested business interest in making America's health care system better. I propose that they be organized into regional depositories and claims processors, with the authority to review the documentation of the providers with the intent to pay, not deny. The legal authority of Fox v Bowen (due process of law) must be vigorously followed. Budgeting for cash flow and rate setting should also be administered by the private sector.

The same companies doing the claims processing can also do the rate setting. Premiums would be individualized and based on each insured person's ongoing health profile. Discounts for fitness, nutritional compliance, screening, and pursuit of health preservation life styles would be substantial. The universal policy would be capped each year as a percent of GNP, and plans for the elimination of the waste in the system would be quantified and used to stay on budget.

Waste patrol according to Deming

Current business practices in health care lend themselves to being hidden on the profit and loss (P/L) statements, and the cost of intangibles are never line itemed. However, the cost of intangible waste is not identified on those statements. In the typical nursing home, staff turnover averages 89% or $250,000 per year in recruiting and retraining costs. Each patient receives 15 to 20 medications daily, based on phone orders from physicians that never see the patient. 50% of patients in nursing homes are re-hospitalized more than four times per year. 50% of staff habitually do not show up on weekends and patients are on their own most of the time. 75% of patients on Medicaid in nursing homes were self—reliant all their lives, until they were put on spend down of their assets and became a ward of the State.

Liability insurance has escalated to the point of being prohibitive in some states. Some organizations are paying upwards to $1 million dollars per year per facility for liability insurance. Most nursing homes have up to 20% excess capacity and do not know how to properly bill for the medical services they are providing to Medicare patients. Lost billings account for $250,000 to $500,000 per facility.

Solution: What if that waste were highlighted by each provider as the object of their management teams to eliminate, or at least reduce each year for the betterment of an aging society? The staff could then be rewarded a percent of the savings and stop being part of the problem. The result would be an end to turnovers, absenteeism, irresponsibility, and theft. What if the line staff were trained and expected to do the right thing when it came to problem resolution at the lowest level? We could save billions, have more fun, and be a better society if employees were listened to and given the latitude to improve their operations.

Here's an example. I met a man in Columbus, Ohio one night watching a Bulls game. He was from Waterloo, Iowa, visiting Columbus to give a speech for the U.S. Chamber of Commerce on management. I was there to present a speech for a nursing home convention. Here is his story: "My Company was on the verge of bankruptcy. I did not know what to do to prevent it from going down. It had gotten to me so badly that I decided to just turn it over to the employees and disappear for two weeks. I was running away from the problems. I stayed away for a month. I didn't go near it for 30 days. When I decided to return, I found that the place was still there going strong, and had turned the corner on some of the labor issues. The leader of the employee group told me that it was better because the people were now taking responsibility for their survival, and suggested that I leave again. I left, came back in two months, and things were better yet. Over the next year, I was gone almost all of the time and the business was never better. The bills were getting out, the payables were being paid on time, and the bottom line was positive for the first time in months. To make my story real and believable, I now travel around the country telling business owners that those in the trenches know what to do if you let them do it!"

Therefore, the modern day management solution to health care is to let the problem makers be the problem solvers before the waste gets a chance to materialize.

Politicians create problems so they can solve them

Senator Newt Gingrich and Senator Bob Dole insisted on the decentralization of Medicaid, which put 50 states in a spending chaos. 45 of those states have proclaimed Medicaid their biggest financial problem. Now, Senator Gingrich is back, claiming to transform health care so every person in American can be their own insurance company. The mistake we make is assuming that the political system can solve any social or business problem. They cannot. They make them worse by creating obstacles to efficiency, ineffective regulations that impede quality, committees and study groups of academics, grants to colleges, and universities that have never been in the trenches, proposing incremental band aids.

Solution:

Senator Hillary Clinton and Senator Ted Kennedy also do not have the answer by having the Government control everything. It has to be the best of both Enterprise and Government. Enterprise is good at pursuing a profit using any means and Government is good at taxing those means. Why not have the Government mandate the standardized processes and have businesses carry them out? The objectives and procedures are simple:

Objectives:

1. Standardize the National Health Policy.
2. Make efficient use of computers for modeling the care and tracking the outcomes.
3. Make effective use of people resources by managing each person's personal resources for the preservation of their health and the prevention of chronic disease.
4. Allow Medicare and Medicaid programs to be the true safety nets for catastrophic episodes.
5. Make coverage for the uninsured and under insured possible by eliminating the hidden costs (waste).Use Six Sigma processes to eliminate the waste.

Procedures:

1. Eliminate the costly and ineffective enforcement mechanisms that exist. Turn inspectors into Six Sigma consultants

who find the providers doing something right, and let the problem makers be the problem solvers.

2. Allow provider associations to police their members by providing case management systems to all providers who can communicate the same language. Make the processes fully integrated with the regulatory imperatives for cost effectiveness and quality control.

3. Set up a national Department of Quality Control, replacing the current ineffective Centers for Medicare and Medicaid (CMS) organization. Allow the Social Security Administration to enforce the National Health Policy.

4. Take the budgeting for health care away from the Office of Management and Budget. Instead, have private companies who administer the collection and disbursement of the premiums, propose the national health care budget. The companies would be responsible for setting the premiums for all Americans and managing the savings accounts for each individual.

5. Focus America on fitness, nutrition and health preservation as a national priority. The goal by the year 2015 will be to match future health care costs with health care savings accounts, based on age, health profiles and earnings from investments.

6. Redirect the medical, nursing, and therapy schools to teach the pursuit of outcome approaches for the purpose of solving the malpractice insurance escalation. Insure that quality of life is based on health preservation, not on the pursuit of treatment. Medicine needs to be a deductive process, based on evidence of causation and projected outcomes.

Performance Based Payment

Measurable restorative goals for each problem exhibited by the patient will establish the platform for performance based payment. The deductive care planning processes replacing inductive "rule out theory" and "least invasive treatment" strategies will convert the practitioners to problem solvers. Currently, the primary physician's hands are tied by the reimbursement methods.

The RVU (Relative Value Units) system is an averaging payment method that pays for treatment, not outcomes. This is also true of the DRG (Diagnosis Related Groups) system for hospitals, the RUG's (Resource Utilization Groups) system for skilled nursing facilities, the OASIS (Outcome and Assessment Information Set) system for home care and OPPS (Outpatient Prospective Payment System) for outpatient services. All of these payment methods must be supported by regulatory provisos and threats, which encourage up-coding and hunting for the best rate, rather than the best outcome.

In 2005, physicians were paid $211 billion dollars for their share of the expanding pie. Hospitals received $616 billion and nursing homes $121 billion. Why isn't this plenty of money? Why don't we have plenty of people resources? Because we have no standardized system for planning the use of resources and no measuring stick for assessing the effectiveness of the workers' performance.

Solution—SHIFT the Paradigm to Self-Health

Pay for the outcome for each problem in the plan of care for each discipline. The use of case management software to blueprint the care and plan the duration of the care can also become the basis for payment. The use of computerized models of care based on medical diagnosis, nursing diagnosis, interventions and goals can be used to direct the care. Hold the clinicians accountable for their time and motion, so the costs and quality are controlled, and have that be the basis for paying them.

Savings will be generated by focusing the care on results, not on payment. Practice, then, can drive reimbursement for the first time ever. The clinicians can be paid fairly, timely, and without fear of reprisal. There will be no need for the extension fraud and abuse infrastructure that now exist, which claim to have caught most of the health care professionals plotting on how to game the system. Wouldn't it be refreshing to catch the providers doing something right for a change?

In conclusion, better care for less money must be the #1 priority, so we can insure everyone in America. This is not only admirable, it is a necessity for an aging population that is still dependent on its medicine to survive. Hopefully, that dependence will change to health preservation and prevention of chronic disease so that we can all afford retirement. By shifting the paradigm to (SHIFT) Self-Health Insurance Funding Trusts withheld from each employees paycheck and allow them to decide when and where to spend it on their disease prevention and health preservation program.

CHANGE—Niagara Falls and the Health Care Crisis

Niagara Falls is one of the wonders of the world. Billions of gallons of water per day (actually 1 million gallons per second) pour unrelenting and uncontrolled into the churning fray below. Sounds like health care . . . millions of dollars per hour ($2 trillion dollars divided by 31,536,000 seconds in a year = $63,419 per second or $3,805,140 per hour) pours unrelenting and uncontrolled into the churning fray below.

What if we had to change the direction of Niagara Falls because it was flooding everything in sight downstream? "Impossible, improbable, unnatural, never can be done." This is what they say about changing the direction of health care . . . impossible, improbable, unnatural, never can be done even though it is flooding everything downstream with runaway costs, inefficiency and poor quality.

Why would you want to change the direction of Niagara Falls? Currently the Falls generates 4 million kilowatts of energy. What if you knew that by changing direction you could improve its output by 2 million kilowatts and avoid a near hurricane force catastrophe? That would certainly give you incentive to try.

While it's not a likely occurrence, changing the direction of Niagara Falls would be far from impossible. All you have to do is turn off the faucet. Find the source of water and shut it down. That would involve placing a dam on the mouth of the Niagara River. Then reroute the flow of water from north to south to west to east. In a few days the Falls would be more powerful than ever and headed in a completely different direction.

The same is true of health care costs. To get this powerful force moving in a different direction we could just turn off the faucet. We could shut down the Government funding and reroute it so that it stops paying for treatment and starts paying for outcomes. Then the providers could no longer claim that what they do is an Art Form: that it is an uncontrollable force of nature, unrelenting in its limitless possibilities. This modification in the flow of spending resources would force the artists to paint by the numbers they demand for payment.

The numbers would be generated by a template connecting diagnosis to cause to problem to intervention to outcome. This is a logical sequencing of the medical process. It involves the physician, the institution, the nurse, the therapist, the social worker, the support staff and the systems network it takes to process the data.

Why would we want to do that? I have 2 million good reasons. In the more than 130 nursing homes I have turned around financially by instituting outcome-based care they sent home an average of ten additional patients per month. If all 16,000 American nursing homes would do the same we would send 2 million patients home a year with a potential savings to the government (from drastically reduced Medicare and Medicaid costs) of nearly $99 billion. (Each day a patient does not need government health care dollars saves an average of $135. Multiply that number by 2 million and you get $270 million dollars a day, times 365 days.)

Nothing is difficult if you decide you have to do it. America's total nursing home capacity—our number of available beds—is 1.9 million. According to the American Association for Homes and Service for the Aging (AAHSA) by 2020, 12 million Americans will need nursing home care. How can we manage that capacity if we don't change course?

A MODERN PARABLE (a reprint)—AN ANALOGY ABOUT THE VALUE OF CHANGING COURSE

A Japanese company (Toyota) and an American company (General Motors) decided to have a canoe race on the Missouri River. Both teams practiced long and hard to reach their peak performance before the race.

On the big day, the Japanese won by a mile.

The Americans, very discouraged and depressed, decided to investigate the reason for the crushing defeat. A management team made up of senior management was formed to investigate and recommend appropriate action. Their conclusion was the Japanese had 8 people rowing and 1 person steering, while the American team had 8 people steering and 1 person rowing.

Feeling a deeper study was in order; American management hired a consulting company and paid them a large amount of money for a second opinion. They advised, of course, that too many people were steering the boat, while not enough people were rowing.

Not sure of how to utilize that information, but wanting to prevent another loss to the Japanese, the rowing team's management structure was totally reorganized to 4 steering supervisors, 3 area steering superintendents and 1 assistant superintendent steering manager.

They also implemented a new performance system that would give the 1 person rowing the boat greater incentive to work harder. It was called the 'Rowing Team Quality First Program,' with meetings, dinners and free pens for the rower. There was discussion of getting new paddles, canoes and other equipment, extra vacation days for practices and bonuses.

The next year the Japanese won by two miles.

Humiliated, the American management laid off the rower for poor performance, halted development of a new canoe, sold the paddles, and canceled all capital investments for new equipment. The money saved was distributed to the Senior Executives as bonuses and the next year's racing team was out-sourced to India

Sad, but oh so true! Here's something else to think about: Ford has spent the last thirty years moving all its factories out of the US, claiming they can't make money paying American wages. Toyota has spent the last thirty years building more than a dozen plants inside the US. The last quarter's results: Toyota makes 4 billion in profits while Ford racked up 9 billion in losses. Ford folks are still scratching their heads. *Perhaps they don't see the value in changing course!*

(Or maybe we just need the Japanese to run our health care system)

How can we shut off the faucet for the Health Care Falls? Shut down the current pay 4 treatment systems and restart it as pay 4

Jerry Rhoads

performance using with economic incentives to accomplish moral incentives.

1) Stop paying for a diagnosis (DRG's) in hospitals
2) Stop paying for room and board and a treatment (RUG's) in nursing homes
3) Stop paying for a prescription in medicine (RVU's)
4) Stop paying for emergency room visits (OPPS)

How would we reroute the cash flow for patient care?

1) Start paying bonuses for outcomes in hospitals

   a. Lowering dependency on medications
   b. Reducing dependency on chemicals
   c. Improving nutritional knowledge
   d. Developing a plan for preserving health
   e. Counseling on weight reduction, obesity, diabetic tendencies
   f. Consulting on preventing chronic diseases

2) Pay Physicians bonuses for

   a. Lowering dependence on medications
   b. Counseling on weight management
   c. Consulting on fitness training regimen
   d. Developing a care plan for preventing chronic diseases
   e. Providing screening and testing services at office

3) Pay nursing homes bonuses for

   a. Home discharges
   b. Health preservation services
   c. Counsel on weight management
   d. Consult on fitness

 e. Providing screening and testing services at the facility
 f. Add-ons for

  i. Physical rehab
  ii. Occupational rehab
  iii. Social rehab
  iv. Speech and swallowing rehab
  v. ADL Restorative programs

   1. Bathing
   2. Dressing
   3. Eating
   4. Grooming
   5. Walking
   6. Communicating

This is Pay 4 Performance and Evidence Based Medicine personified. HHS wants this and they will have it. All we need to do is shut off the way the cash is currently flowing and redirect the way we spend the money. Obviously, we need to do something to improve not only the results but also the effectiveness of the cost.

Why will this sell? It is a win-win for all the stakeholders:

- Hospitals will be paid well and timely for being the crisis center . . .
- Physicians will be paid well and timely for being the gatekeeper for preserving health and preventing chronic illnesses.
- Nursing homes will be paid for transitioning the elderly back into community based programming
- Home and emergency care will be the safety net for dealing with episodic interventions.
- Government purchasers get results and prevention of high cost hospitalizations and the dangers of poly pharmacy.

Jerry Rhoads

- Patients receive counseling, consulting and preventive services for preserving health and dealing with crisis care at the lowest cost alternative . . . home and outpatient services.

Redirecting this mighty flow of cash will produce some mighty powerful results.

THE LAST WORD

Making the paradigm shift from the Red Zone to the Self-Health culture is dependent on individual commitment to changing personal beliefs about guiding their own health not depending on pills and chemicals to do it for them. Our Government is leading us to believe that they can set up the mechanism for managing the health of populations using money as the motivator and the providers of the health care services as the catalyst to mass better habits. This has failed in the past and will fail in the future . . . the process is a science not a political debate on cost and how to use incomes to produce desired outcomes. It is each individual's responsibility to better their own heath by changing their bad living habits to their natural state which is managing their own diet, time usage and commitment to improving their own health for living longer and better.

Analyzing the list of the 100 oldest people in the world and the profiles of the Baby Boomers demonstrates the differences in the life styles of females versus males. There are only 5 males on the list of the 100 oldest and other 95 are females. Not surprising if you go into a nursing home and see mostly females. However, we also realize that that mix is changing every day due to the changing culture for men and women. Smoking or not smoking and stressful living or not gainfully employed are probably being the most significant factors. So we need to benefit from what we have experienced:

- Stop smoking Start deep breathing
- Stop sitting Start getting out of the chair
- Stop gripping Start finding your talent and a job
- Stop Bidding time Start yourself on a mission
- Stop procrastinating Start your venture
- Stop worrying about money Start planning for another career
- Stop Riding rather than walking Start an exercise program
- Stop being negative Start meditating on happiness
- Stop Killing yourself Start living longer and better

Our society does not move its brain and body enough. It is showing in the numbers of over-weight people but more importantly it is permeating to our youngsters. No longer do we have a lean and mean look to our youth . . . also the work ethic seems to be different . . . the values are different . . . the foul language has escalated . . . the use of texting, sexting, videos, violence, porn, teen pregnancy, drugs, alcoholism, etc. are all signs of a deteriorating society.

Is all lost? Hell no if we decide to make changes in our social mores, habits and values . . . our leaders need to emphasize this, not fighting about issues and dividing us on social problems that the constitution has already decided:

- Abortion has a connection to human rights as stated in the Fifth and Fourteenth Amendments . . . the expectant mother has the right to decide whether she will be ready and able to sustain a life
- Same sex marriage has a connection to the Fifth and Fourteenth Amendments giving each citizen the right to freedom of choice and life as defined by individual's capability to sustain life

- Gay rights has a connection to the Fifth and Fourteenth Amendments giving each citizen the right to choose a mate
- Civil rights has a connection to the Fifth and Fourteenth Amendments giving each color, creed, religious beliefs, age, gender the right to choose a life style at their own individual risk
- Health and welfare of the citizens are not a right but a privilege under the Fifth and Fourteenth Amendments that states the each individual is free to choose their life style and are responsible for their own health and welfare needs

All is lost if we are not dealing with social problems that need to be addressed, not with more laws, but with leadership initiatives:

- Reducing the size of government
- Having all Americans participate in governance
- Reducing the size of the cache of our weapons of mass destruction
- Promote peace rather than liberty as defined by our values
- Lead the world to better health and a prosperous standard of living

All too many people take our great country for granted and expect someone else to make the decisions on their lives . . . not good . . . that is the way democracy is replaced by Government for socialistic reasons that are in reality an erosion of our individual freedoms as stated in the Constitution. We are at a juncture in our history where the individual needs to be the focus not the greater good . . . we all must take responsibility for our own future, wellness, standard of living and happiness. And elect leaders who believe in the enterprising nature of Americans that is being quashed by too many laws, law makers and money driven values. If we are not willing to stand up for our country we are willing to fall for anything proposed by a few control freaks. Not good!

BABY BOOMERS
IN THE SELF- HEALTH END ZONE
BY JERRY RHOADS

The Boomers are here
The impact is fear
After the end of the Great war in '45
Brides and Grooms came alive

Boosting the pregnancy rate
Opening the baby gate
Christening 77 million by '65
Putting us in economic overdrive

Starting in 2005 they want to retire
Long before they expire
Maxing out their social security checks
Leaving entitlements as fiscal wrecks

Paying their share of tax bills if wealthy
Believing that Medicare will keep them healthy
Being the driving force of the Great Society
What they were promised is impropriety

However like much in today's politics
The Boomers will demand and vote for a fix
Finding no equity in money-tics
Like the ride of Paul Revere

Then when all is said and done
Those moving from the Red Zone
Into that wonderful Self-Health End Zone
Will have won

"Never fear The Boomers are here"

Appendix I

CAN WE AFFORD A SELF-HEALTH AMERICA? The following is a reproduction of the proposed Obama budget for the period 2013 to 2022 as published in the Office of Management Budget for the federal government. It has not been approved, nor has any budget been approved by the House of Representatives since Obama took office.

Table S—1. 2013 Budget totals (in billions of dollars and as a percent of GDP)

	2011	2012	2013	2014	2015	2016	2017	2018	2019	2020	2021	2022	2013-17	2013-22
Budget totals in billions of dollars:														
Receipts	$2,303	$2,469	$2,902	$3,215	$3,450	$3,680	$3,919	$4,153	$4,379	$4,604	$4,857	$5,115	$17,167	$40,274
Outlays	3,603	3,796	3,803	3,883	4,060	4,329	4,532	4,728	5,004	5,262	5,537	5,820	20,607	46,959
Deficit	-1,300	-1,327	-901	-668	-610	-649	-612	-575	-626	-658	-681	-704	-3,440	-6,684
Debt held by the public	$10,128	$11,578	$12,637	$13,445	$14,198	$14,980	$15,713	$16,404	$17,137	$17,897	$18,678	$19,486		
Debt net of financial assets	9,170	10,467	11,358	12,023	12,633	13,281	13,894	14,469	15,095	15,753	16,433	17,137		
Gross domestic product	14,959	15,602	16,335	17,156	18,178	19,261	20,369	21,444	22,421	23,409	24,427	25,488		
Budget totals as a percent of GDP:														
Receipts	15%	16%	18%	19%	19%	19%	19%	19%	20%	20%	20%	19%	19%	19%
Outlays	24%	24%	23%	22%	22%	22%	22%	22%	22%	22%	22%	22%	22%	22%
Deficit	8.7%	8.5%	5.5%	3.9%	3.4%	3.4%	3.0%	2.7%	2.8%	2.8%	2.8%	2.8%	3.8%	3.3%
Debt held by the public	67.7%	74.2%	77.4%	78.4%	78.1%	77.8%	77.1%	76.5%	76.4%	76.5%	76.5%	76.5%		
Debt net of financial assets	61.3%	67.1%	69.5%	70.1%	69.5%	69.0%	68.2%	67.5%	67.3%	67.3%	67.3%	67.2%		

OBMA'S PROPOSED BUDGET FOR 2013

1. Budgeting over $1.3 trillion to $700 billion every year to totaling $6.6 trillion accumulated deficit by 2022
2. Total debt of $20 trillion budgeted by 2022
3. Receipts 15 percent to 19 percent of GNP by 2022
4. Outlays 24 percent to 22 percent of GNP every year to 2022
5. Debt held by public 76.5 percent of GNP by 2022
6. Debt net of financial assets 67.2 percent by 2022
7. Annual interest of $800 billion by 2022
8. Does not factor in the escalation of healthcare costs of $1 trillion per year due to the baby boomers and Obama Care impact on Medicaid, half of which is shifted to the states' bloated budgets
9. Source: published federal budget proposal for the next ten years

Department of Health and Human Services Budget
Healthcare administration federal level (in millions of dollars)
Actual 2011, estimate 2012-2013

	2011	2012	2013
Administration on Children and Families (ACF)	$17,210	$16,489	$16,194
Administration on Aging	1,497	1,471	1,978
General Departmental Management	655	474	306
Office of Civil Rights	41	41	39
Office of the National Coordinator for Health Information Technology	42	16	26
Program Level (non-add)	61	61	66
Office of Medicare Hearing and Appeals	70	72	84
Public Health and Social Services Emergency Fund	675	568	642
Office of Inspector General	50	50	59
All other	51	43	37
Subtotal, Discretionary Budget Authority	$76,472	$76,186	$76,446

Discretionary Changes in Mandatory Programs *(non-add in 2012):* Children's Health Insurance Program Reauthorization Act of 2009—			
Performance Bonuses		*-6,368*	-6,706
Consumer Operated and Oriented Plan (CO-OP) Program			-400
High Risk Pool			44
ACF—13			
Subtotal, Discretionary changes in mandatory programs		*-6,724*	-6,719
Total, Discretionary budget authority	76,472	76,186	69,727
Discretionary Cap Adjustment: Program Integrity			270 299
Rescission of Balances of Funds Provided by P.L. 111 -32 -1,259—			
Total, Discretionary outlays	86,528	84,160	80,605
Mandatory Outlays: Medicare Baseline Outlays	480,202	479,338	528,556
Legislative proposal			-4,807
Medicaid and Children's Health Insurance Program (CHIP)			
Existing law	283,597	265,011	292,856
Legislative proposal		155	190
All other Existing law	41,007	43,057	42,901
Legislative proposal			1 639
Total, Mandatory outlays	$804,806	$787,777	$860,335

Obama Care 2013 to 2022 budget for regulatory enforcement employing 16,000 more IRS agents to police the penalties and 15,000 Recovery Audit Contractors (RAC) to find alleged fraud and abuse among providers of care.

1. $860 million for program administration at federal level
2. Another $250 million at the state level
3. $1 billion per year for enforcement of Medicare and Medicaid

4. Budget includes numerous reforms for savings
5. Source published federal budget proposal for the next ten years

The Monopsony Game (Government controlled Board Game) demonstrating the power of the Government in our lives is available through the American Enterprise Party web site.

Department of Defense (in millions of dollars)
Actual 2011, estimate 2012-2013 spending

Discretionary Base Budget Authority:	2011	2012	2013
Military personnel	$137,046	$141,819	$135,113
Operation and maintenance	192,649	197,198	208,744
Procurement	103,909	104,464	98,823
Research, development, test, and Evaluation	75,733	71,375	69,408
Military construction	14,768	11,367	9,572
Family housing	1,819	1,683	1,651
Revolving and management funds	2,348	2,641	2,123
Subtotal, discretionary base budget authority	528,272	530,547	525,434
Discretionary cap adjustment:			
Overseas contingency operations (OCO)	158,753	115,083	88,482
Total, discretionary budget authority (base and OCO)	687,025	645,630	613,916
Total, discretionary outlays (base and OCO)	673,848	682,995	666,159
Total, mandatory outlays	4,226	5,260	6,721
Total, outlays	$678,074	$688,255	$672,880
Credit activity			
Direct loan disbursements:			
Family housing improvement direct loan financing account	309	202	195
Total, direct loan disbursements	309	202	195

1 The Balanced Budget and Emergency Deficit Control Act of 1985 (BBEDCA), as amended by the Budget Control Act of 2011, limits—or caps—budget authority available for discretionary programs each year through 2021. Section 251(b)(2) of BBEDCA authorizes certain adjustments to the caps after the enactment of appropriations. Amounts in 2011 are not so designated but are shown for comparability purposes.

Footnotes:

1. Assumes Overseas Contingency Operations assumes troops being withdrawn from Iraq and Afghanistan
2. Assumes savings will be used to offset sequestered defense cuts
3. Budget includes numerous reforms for savings
4. Source: published federal budget proposal for the next ten years

Gross national income, $15.23 trillion PPP dollars, current prices, 2011

The U.S. budget deficit hit a record $1.4 trillion (£877 billion) in the year ended September 30, 2012 U.S. Congress estimates say. The deficit was equal to 9.9 percent of gross domestic product (GDP)—more than treble the 2008 level and the highest since the end of World War II. Source: per the World Bank

On the Other Hand Can America Afford Being Unhealthy? If not, how can individuals make a difference rather than expecting the healthy taxpayers to continue to pay for unhealthy taxpayers regardless of their actions and habits? It isn't working now and putting the Government in charge removes success and a healthy nation totally out of the individuals' grasp. The end zone is within our grasp if we SHIFT THE PARADIGM TO SELF PRESERVATION HABITS AND THINKING!

APPENDIX II

How Politicians and Regulators
Make It Impossible for Small Businesses
to Create and Procreate

IS AMERICA BECOMING THE NEXT VERSION OF THE HUNGER GAMES?

**According to Suzanne Collin's trilogy "Hunger Games",
after the demise of the Games and the revolution against
the totalitarian CAPITOL Government for the sake of
humanity; there was to be Peace on Earth.** "The questions are
just beginning. The arenas have been completely destroyed, the
memorials built, there are no more Hunger Games. But they teach
about them at school, and the girl knows we played a role in them.
The boy will know in a few years. How can I tell them about a
world without frightening them to death? My children, who take
the words of the song for granted:

> Deep in the meadow, under the willow,
> A bed of grass, a soft green pillow
> Lay down your head, and close your sleepy eyes
> And when again they open, the sun will rise.

> Here it's safe, here it's warm
> Here the daisies guard you from every harm
> Here your dreams are sweet and tomorrow brings them true
> Here is the place where I love you."

Thanks to Suzanne Collins' version of how ordinary victims of oppression can deny the Capitol's totalitarian use of fear, indulgence and deprivation for inhumane control . . . by taking what we learn in the Hunger Games we now have the opportunity to avoid that same struggle by peacefully replacing our government's bureaucratic and regulatory approach to controlling life with common folk sense for an enterprising rewarding life. But this requires that the Enterprise be a third alternative to our current Two Party Oppressive (Regulatory) Games. "Give us enterprise or give us debt" that is our challenge.

"Big Government Rides Again: a True Story of Government Corrupt Intrusion into Enterprise," by Jerry Rhoads

Jerry Rhoads' Position Paper On Regulators Retaliation Against the Paradigm Shift to Deductive Health Care Economics . . . following is my personal experience of calculated retaliation for implementing outcome based payment and re-enforcement surveys . . . November 2011 in Muscatine and Washington Iowa.

Small Business Loses Again to Big Government

Local nursing care center fights back. State of Iowa regulators retaliate against All-American Care of Washington. Facts: an entrepreneur, Jerry Rhoads, is from Iowa originally. He, his wife, and his son have returned to Iowa on a mission. It is to change the paradigm for caring for aging Americans from the traditional nursing home to a restorative care center.

They purchased the Muscatine Care Center in September 2009 and have converted it to the Restorative Model of Care. The Restorative Model, invented by the Rhoads family, versus institutional care, is like night and day. We all know what the institutions have not been able to do. The Restorative Model, on the other hand, restores the whole person to their highest level of physical, mental, social, and spiritual functioning.

The Rhoads have proven in two-and-a-half short years, at their Muscatine facility, that this model works where the institutional model has not. Using this approach, the Rhoads family has taken an old institutional business, invested $400,000 in renovation to restore dignity, and converted antiquated systems to modern computer and security systems to bring quality of care and life to Iowans.

This approach has resulted in many more of the elderly being restored and returned home (55% to be exact). There are fewer being sent to the hospital ER or beds (less than 17% to be exact), and there is reduced dependency on prescription drugs (33% fewer pills). These are the dramatic results at the All-American Care of Muscatine.

The Rhoads family then purchased another failing nursing home in Washington, Iowa, for the purpose of doing the same extreme makeover there. The community is thrilled to have the facility back in the business community. To date, $400,000 has been invested in the renovations on top of the purchase price, and four months later, the facility is becoming respectable.

Now comes the bad news. As in the Muscatine conversion, the inherited policies, procedures, systems, and methods have to be upgraded or changed. Staff are now in a team environment with specific uniforms (nurses in white, not scrubs) and have accountability systems directing them. Many don't want change and leave or are terminated. In Muscatine, over 150 employees were replaced or hired for new positions until the right professionals were in place. In the process, the business doubled its revenues and created fifty new jobs.

The same process is being implemented in Washington, and then a disgruntled employee called the State of Iowa Department of Inspections and Appeals hotline with a five-part complaint, namely:

1. The building is too cold
2. The staff are sleeping at night
3. Incontinent patients are not changed timely
4. Baths are not given timely
5. Inadequate supervision

Under the enforcement rules followed by the State of Iowa, the provider is guilty until proven innocent. The following is the insanity that small business faces with Big Government:

1. Anyone, any time can call the state hotline with any trumped up violation . . . particularly from a former or current disgruntled employee.
2. State must by regulations investigate on site every complaint.
3. The complainant does not have to inform the facility, before calling the state, giving the facility a chance to correct this allegation.
4. The state sends a complaint surveyor into the facility unannounced and holds them hostage for days at a time.
5. By regulation, they do not have to inform the facility of who complained, why they complained, and the facility's right to defend themselves.
6. The surveyor is to focus on the complaint stated in the phone call, unless they detect noncompliance elsewhere . . . and they always do.

7. Violation detection is the objective of the surveyor . . . dig and you will certainly find dirt . . . and they generally do.
8. A report of deficiencies is then issued from the state DIA office after the surveyor givers a noncommittal cursory report to the facility regarding findings before exiting the facility.
9. The higher-ups in Des Moines assign scope and severity codes to each violation with no cross examination or testimony from the facility; and establish punitive allegations and fines while holding Medicare/Medicaid reimbursement for new admissions, forcing the facility into an appeal. The presumed violations are then posted on the DIA website as final, for all to see, two days after the notice is sent to the provider.
10. The facility is given ten days from the date the surprises hit the provider's fax machine or e-mail to garner a defense, if any. Typically, the facility knuckles under and allows this to go on their eternal record, which can be used against them in later surveys.

Now does that sound like due process of law and compliant with the Administrative Procedures Act? No . . . that is why I am dredging up this issue. When the state descends on us that way, it isn't right and is not improving care one inch . . . and has not in the thirty years I have been exposed to it. It is insanity, working overtime.

Yes, nursing homes, for the most part, have been despicable, smelly, and depressing institutions. Most are owned and operated by owners and investors who never go there. (The owners of Muscatine had never been there in thirty years). Real estate has been the focus of the builders, operators, and well-meaning entrepreneurs. But the real business is the restoration of the elderly and disabled to their highest level of functioning so they can return home. That is the stated objective of the Medicare law that is violated daily by the federal government's interpretation of what they will not pay for. Typically, the elderly and disabled do not get their entitled 100 days per spell of illness in skilled nursing facilities because of Big Government's denial of payment to the providers. Fear is their tactic, punishment is their method.

The average coverage period for a post hospital Medicare patient is twenty-five to thirty days, if therapy is involved . . . with no extended coverage for skilled nursing restoring function, emotional stability, socialization, and performing home inspections.

Now to the point of this position paper on how Big Government kills small business. On January 25 (three months after All-American Care took over ownership of Washington Care Center), a complaint surveyor came unannounced with the five-part complaint. And over the next three weeks, off and on (January 26, 30, 31 and February 6 and 7, 2012) he dug in to find everything he could through his five-part porthole. The reason for the investigation is not the issue, even though it wastes everyone's time on unsubstantiated complaints.

In this case, three of the five parts were not substantiated but are on the record books. The other two resulted in F-tag 309 and 323 "G" and an "E" severity code 320 being assessed . . . the G level violations automatically generate fines and withholding of reimbursement until the revisit clears the tags. In this case, the state officials went back to a previous owner's survey results seven months prior and decided to treble the fines . . . so now the $5,000 becomes $15,000, plus $3,000 for lesser violations, plus $300 per day if the plan of care is not timely. All this gets published, and for all they care, we could be forced out of business before we can finish our conversion.

This does not follow the Administrative Procedures Act or the rule of law. And according to administrative rule of law, the providers are allowed due process for contesting allegations and fines.

However, all we are allowed is an Informal Dispute Review (IDR) with very strict limitations as to what we can present.

And now for the worst of it . . . All-American Care is using video security cameras in its facilities, as a quality assurance tool, to be able to view staff, patients, visitors, and surveyors activities for the safely of all. Sounds like the right-thing intention. Well, in this case, it hung us with our own rope because the surveyor got wind of it and viewed twenty-four hours' worth of data over an eight-hour period to look at what was going on while he was not there. It then became his tool for incriminating and misinterpreting an incident he wasn't even there to investigate . . . falls in the secured unit.

The first incident happened in our locked secure unit for demented and Alzheimer's patients. A behavior problem patient, who had been banging her head on the wall of her room and ripping the curtains down, was viewed on the video stumbling down the hall toward the nursing station, holding up her arms, apparently talking to the ceiling tile.

She stops and proceeds, and then walks backward until she stumbles and falls backward, hits the base of her head, rubs it with her hand, rolls over against the wall, and remains there. The patient's documented history is of misbehaving and having a habit of lying on the floor in her room or in her closet and had done this at least three times during the previous two days. In this unit, that is acceptable behavior and is not to be construed automatically as a fall.

So the surveyor viewed the video and requested that they see the whole twenty-four-hour period. Kip Rhoads, the director of Operations, agrees to let him view the recorded data, assuming that it would absolve the facility of any wrongdoing . . . instead he calculated that it had been forty-eight minutes before anyone responded to what he was now labeling a fall.

Two CNAs were observed coming down the hall and glancing over at the patient thinking she was all right, and then decided to check her . . . rolled her over, and lifted her to her feet. There was no blood, no injury noted, and the staff assumed she was all right.

The patient was some 100 feet down the hall from the nursing station and the testimony from the two staff that were there was they just thought she was doing what she usually was doing . . . lying on the floor. Later, a different CNA found blood in her hair and a laceration to the right side of her head. She was taken to the hospital Emergency Room and the laceration closed and stapled. Later, she returned from ER that day and was then discharged to the hospital psycho ward and never returned.

From that point in the video examination, the surveyor began investigating other falls in the rest of facility and cited additional deficiencies that resulted in a cumulative of two "G" level violations.

The violation became as follows:

1. Any patient on the floor constitutes a fall.(patient has the right to lay on the floor)
2. Facility staff neglected to respond to the patient's injury (even though they did not know of her injury).
3. With a known fall, a nurse must assess the patient's condition for injury, call the family and doctor . . . then perform prescribed interventions. This was not done in this circumstance and constitutes, according to the surveyor, a life-threatening event that requires a self-report to the state and documentation in the patient's record with an incident report of the injury and outcome.

We accept responsibility for not responding timely to the patient lying on the floor . . . however, the staff did respond after deciding that she should be checked and the Director of Nursing testified to the surveyor that they did not know this was a fall but acceptable behavior, and the only way the surveyor was able to determine the response time was by clocking the video and staying another three days viewing more video and assessing more allegations and fines.

He dug into bathing schedules and documentation and asserted that a patient had not been bathed for nine days but did not accept testimony that this patient habitually refuses baths and was given sponge or bed baths in the interim. It was not the facility's procedure to record bed baths on the bath sheet. The very statement that we did not bath a patient for nine days is not factual nor can the surveyor prove differently.

Summary:

1. New providers are expected to meet a higher standard of care than the previous provider.
2. By rule, the video, being a Quality Assurance tool, is to be off-limits to the surveyors. We were led to believe that he was wanting to absolve us of any wrongdoing; whereas, he used it to incriminate and entrap us for the sake of justifying his three weeks at our facility.
3. A double "G" level of violations with treble damages is the worst scenario for a Quality Assurance tool that we allowed the surveyor to use, in good faith, leaving us to deal with the next bureaucratic step up to an IDR . . . which warns us that we are not to contest the methods of the survey, the fines, or the allegations, unless we have been charged with substandard care.
4. We will appeal and have little legal standing to the enforcement and punitive nature that the regulators charged. We had visions of helping small communities in Iowa to have quality long-term restorative care and do away with the institutional model . . . but is looks like Big Government wins again.

The Rule of Law

The doctrine of the rule of law dictates that government must be conducted according to law. Judges have identified three essential elements of the Constitution which were indicative of the rule of law:

1. Absence of arbitrary power
2. Equality before the law
3. The Constitution is a result of the ordinary law of the land

Administrative Procedures Act

Standard of Judicial Review

The APA requires that in order to set aside agency action not subject to formal trial-like procedures, the court must conclude that the regulation is "arbitrary and capricious, an abuse of discretion, or otherwise not in accordance with the law."[8] However, Congress may further limit the scope of judicial review of agency actions by including such language in the organic statute. To set aside formal rule-making or formal adjudication whose procedures are trial-like (*see* APA, 5 U.S.C 556[9]-557[10]), a different standard of review allows courts to question agency action more strongly. For these more formal actions, agency decisions must be supported by "substantial evidence"[11] after the court reads the "whole record,"[12] which can be thousands of pages long.

Unlike arbitrary and capricious review, substantial evidence review gives the courts leeway to consider whether an agency's factual and policy determinations were warranted in light of all the information before the agency at the time of decision. Accordingly, arbitrary and capricious review is understood to be more deferential to agencies than substantial evidence review. Arbitrary and capricious review allows the agency's decisions to stand as long as an agency can give a reasonable explanation for its decision based on the information it had at the time. In contrast, the courts tend to look much harder at decisions resulting from trial-like procedures because those agency procedures resemble actual trial court procedures, but the Article III of the Constitution reserves the judicial powers for actual courts. Accordingly, courts are strict under the substantial evidence standard when agencies act like courts because being strict gives courts final say, preventing agencies from using too much judicial power, in violation of the doctrine of separation of powers.

The separation of powers doctrine is less of an issue with rule-making not subject to trial-like procedures. Such rule-making gives agencies a lot more leeway in court because it is much more like the legislative process reserved for Congress in Article II. The courts' main role here is ensuring that the agency rules line up with the Constitution and with the agency's statutory commands from Congress. Even if a court finds a rule very unwise, it will stand as long as it is not "arbitrary and capricious, an abuse of discretion, or otherwise not in accordance with the law."

To date, our appeals are still pending, and we are contemplating legal action against the State of Iowa and the Department of Health and Human Services for total disregard of the administrative procedures relating to patient care and due process of law. As I write this on December 18 the surveyors have descended on our Washington, Iowa facility for their enforcement tactics. The question is, are we ever going to get it right or are they going to destroy what is left?

Post Script to a nightmare ending . . . is the latest in a long line of gotcha's for the regulators . . . their latest is we should have done CPR on a dead man . . . punishment for a hair brain allegation that we are still appealing. That is what we get with regulators that have too much authority and no compunction for the human factor.

Appendix **III**

SYNOPSIS OF PATIENT PROTECTION AND
AFFORDABLE CARE ACT—906 PAGES, 217,440 WORDS,
BILLIONS IN GRANTS AND DEMONSTRATION
PROJECTS, PLUS 400 PAGES ON ENFORCEMENT

An e-mail letter to Jerry Rhoads from the future president of the
United States—Senator Barack Obama

Dear Jerry:

Thank you for taking the time to contact me. I
apologize for the delay in my response. Quite frankly, I
was unprepared for the volume of correspondence and
emails I have received since coming to the Senate in
January, 2005 and I am just now finally feeling more
comfortable about my ability to respond in a timely
manner to the thousands of communications I receive
each week from Illinois residents. Your particular
comments about what I should be doing in Washington
to improve access to needed health care are greatly
appreciated.

Thank you for sharing the ecaregiver.com model of
care with me. As it states, we must use methodology
and systems that allow health care providers to more

accurately assess patient needs, provider high quality care, hold health care professionals responsible for outcomes, and create a culture of patient safety.

Be certain that improving and strengthening our nation's health care system is a priority of mine. Thank you for contributing to the debate surrounding this call for improvement.

There should be no question that the President's proposed cuts in Medicare and Medicaid will result in the denial of needed care. To me, these cuts, in a budget that extends the President's tax cuts, reflect a distorted sense of national priorities, and I will fight them.

Sincerely,

Barack Obama
United States Senator

Commentaries by Jerry Rhoads, Author:

After passing the Affordable Health Care Act of 2010, the Obama administration offered the states new ways to improve care, lower costs for Medicaid by *improving care quality for nursing facility residents (however, at a cost of $1 trillion for demonstration projects and another $1 trillion in enforcement of new regulations over the next ten years, health care administration costs will double).*

■ "The Centers of Medicare/Medicaid Services announced today a new initiative to help states improve the quality of care for people in nursing homes. Nearly two-thirds of nursing facility residents are receiving Medicaid benefits, and most are also eligible for Medicare benefits. The CMS Innovation Center in collaboration with the

CMS Medicare-Medicaid Coordination Office will establish a new demonstration focused on reducing preventable inpatient hospitalizations among residents of nursing facilities by providing these individuals with the treatment they need without having to unnecessarily go to a hospital. Hospitalizations are often expensive, disruptive, disorienting, and dangerous for frail elders and people with disabilities and cost Medicare billions of dollars each year. CMS-funded research on Medicare-Medicaid eligible nursing facility residents in 2005 found that almost 40-percent of hospital admissions were preventable, accounting for 314,000 potentially avoidable hospitalizations and $2.6 billion in Medicare expenditures."

■ "Starting in the fall of 2011, CMS will competitively select independent accountable care organizations (ACO's) to partner with and implement evidence-based interventions at interested nursing facilities. These interventions could include using nurse practitioners in nursing facilities, supporting transitions between hospitals and nursing facilities, and implementing best practices to prevent falls, pressure ulcers, urinary tract infections, or other events that lead to poor health outcomes and expensive hospitalizations. Additionally, this initiative supports the administration's Partnership for Patients goal of reducing hospital readmission rates by 20-percent by the end of 2013."

COMMENTARY:

ACO's are a brain child of University demonstration projects and enforcement thereof: Universities and think tanks, which have never operated a health care business, be it a hospital, nursing home, or medical practice, are employed by CMS to tell them what they already have decided . . . keep it administratively simple but complex enough to be ineffective so as to control the flow of dollars to certain providers to keep them quiet. Enforcement is to create the aura of the bad guys in private business ripping off the poor to become rich when the effect it will have is that the poor and aging Americans will be left out in the cold as the dollars are rationed to the younger population. Enforcement will increase the size of the government agency and build on fear as a deterrent . . . so goes health reform . . . no real initiatives to move from an illness—based payment system to a wellness-based payment for outcomes, not incomes.

COMMENTARY:

This 2,500 page giant piece of social legislation is nothing other than a political tactic to keep control over $3 trillion of American taxpayers' money. It throws the private sector under the truck full of perks for universities and think tanks using grants and consulting contracts. Resulting in more social regulations . . . dictated by the federal government, leading us to believe that the vast health care legislation protects us from the horrible insurance companies, the greedy providers, and the ignorance of voters.

In reality, it is one thing to repeal health care reform and another to reform the wasteful spending going on. We pay for illness, not wellness; we pay for pills, not stronger wills; and we pay for incomes, not outcomes. Until we take the authority for determining how to pay away from the bureaucrats, insurance companies, and academics, we will continue to bankrupt the current Medicare, Medicaid, and insurance plans.

AFFORDABLE—NOT

About $1 trillion will be spent over the next decade on research grants to enhance academic and bureaucratic intellectuals' income—takes resources away from improved outcomes. The ACO's will be funded by the Federal Government through capitation formulas that take population groups by age and mathematically determine how much will be spent per capita . . . without regard for quality outcomes with incomes based on cutting the cost per capita to a minimum without regard for the impact aging America will have on the high risk baby boomers.

This takes resources away from true savings programs—the first half of the bill involves a national health care strategy which we need, and the last half wastes enough on enforcement and a wish list to fund the first half.

Who is going to monitor this monster of regulatory and legalese? It will take 16,000 IRS agents, 50,000 bureaucrats and 100,000 attorneys to figure out how to police and how to game the system, while allowing the politicians to control our unhealthy lives.

QUALITY—NOT

Only God knows how the middle class will pay for it: we, the small business owners and taxpayers who already pay FORTY-FOUR different taxes and get no better health care services.

Do we have a commonsense leader in the country that will stop this lawmaking nightmare and start the elimination of imposing and resource wasting laws?

WHAT IT DOES NOT TELL THE TAXPAYER:

1. Impact of rationing out the dollars on the 7,000 Americans per day reaching sixty-five years of age.
2. How 77 million Americans are going to get their benefits when the trust funds will be insolvent by 2021.
3. Puts regulatory enforcement and restricted innovation to government grants in the hands of the bureaucracy. The Department of Health and Human Services has over twenty-five websites that dictate how the money will be rationed out. Many that are based on the premise

of punitive regulatory controls cuts the costs through enforcement; not collaborative and creative enterprise. "You cannot trust the private sector to police its own businesses".

4. Health care payment currently reimburses for illness, not wellness; medications, hospitalizations, tests, re-hospitalizations, ER visits, DRGs, RUGs, RVUs, and OPPS all pay for illness, not wellness.

5. Physicians, hospitals, nurses, therapists, etc., have no standardized processes and think inductively when intervening and establishing care plans.

6. Use of information technology for efficiency requires standardization of terminology and processes to be effective.

7. Best practices will not emerge until we pay for outcomes, not incomes.

8. Why is there only distrust of the private sector to produce better results without infringement on entrepreneurial initiative?

9. It will take creative economic incentives to attain moral incentives. Not 16,000 IRS auditors and 15,000 RAC auditors.

Appendix IV

"The Dorotha C. White Foundation"
"Adopt a Nursing Home Patient" Program

Sharon Rhoads, whose mother Dorotha C. White, for whom the Foundation was formed, died of abuse and neglect in a nursing home. It was not of her choosing and we feel guilty for putting her there. Due to circumstances similar to most families there was no other alternative. Sharon and I are in the business of assisting nursing homes to improve their programming and provide the companionship, emotional counseling, socialization and spiritual services that are so direly needed. With the "adopt a patient program" we are dedicated to avoiding occurrences that befell Dorotha.

Across American we adopt highways, foreign born babies, laws, domestic born babies, foster children, etc. All of this effort is to exercise the heart of a free society, which is to give all human beings a chance at life liberty and the pursuit of happiness. We need to

Restore Elder Pride for the sake of ourselves as we all will need quality of care for our quality of life wishes.

Where this philosophy seems to end is at the threshold of our nursing homes. The institutionalization of the elderly is pandemic and will get much worse with the aging of the baby boomers. I am not an advocate of dumping them back into the community that is not capable or ready to take on such a huge responsibility. My philosophy is that the nursing homes are not homes for the elderly. They are called such and society accepts it as the only alternative. I propose there is another alternative:

1. Recognize that skilled nursing care is not home care . . . it is transitional care.
2. Replace the medical model practiced by physicians, hospitals and nursing homes with the Restorative Model.
3. Encourage community involvement in making the transition.
4. Mandate a reimbursement system that rewards outcomes that improve and restore function.
5. Set up community based programs that assist in the restoration of the elderly back into the community based services . . . "adopt a patient" is that kind of involvement that is needed.

This embraces the body, the mind, the heart and the spirit. This is where the Adopt a Nursing Home Patient Program is critical. Missing in most all nursing homes is the companionship factor, the emotional uplift factor, the socializing factor and the spiritual factor. Why because the staff is not organized to deliver holistic care. It is given lip service at best. We have done studies and literally none of the nursing homes are providing psycho/social programming because they are not being paid for it. This is an alarming fact.

To solve this will take the effort of the community, the politicians, the clinicians, the providers and the families. Under our Adopt a Nursing Home Patient we are dealing with all four factors:

- Companionship—a visit by a real person who is interested in the patient's feelings, needs, problems and hopes will create healing that is not medicinal.

- Emotions—writing a letter to a patient who does not receive mail revitalizes the humanity of knowing someone cares.
- Socialization—currently the patients are grouped around TV's in wheelchairs with no social stimulation . . . why not take a patient to a movie outside the facility and go out to eat and go to the ballgame . . .
- Spiritual stimulation—church can be brought to the patient or the patient can be taken to church. It takes someone doing it.

The Foundation will obtain authorization from the Provider, the family and the State regulators to provide the "adoption of a patient" by a community volunteer to provide the companionship, emotional involvement, socialization and spiritual contact for those who need it, want it and will sign an approval for it.

Why will the provider of care agree to this? The Foundation, on its website will provide free advertising for those providers implementing the "adopt a patient" program. The facility must assist in screening the volunteers coming into their facility and measure the effectiveness of the program. The Foundation will rate the facility using six star criteria before allowing them to participate in the program:

- First Star is for companionship through the use of the adopt a patient program.
- Second Star is for environment . . . cleanliness, no odors, plenty of light, live plants, pets, etc.
- Third Star is for efficient and productive staffing . . . staff organized in teams to provide restorative services and able to show improvements in functioning.
- Fourth Star is for social programs . . . for example reading groups, current events groups, storytelling groups, discussion groups geared to disease process, etc.

* Fifth star is for psychological counseling programs . . . use of group therapies, reducing prescriptions as the alternative to treatment and replacing it with more exercise and better nutritional alternatives.
* Sixth Star is for spiritual involvement of the community churches by allowing the patients to come to outside services.

The Foundation rating as a six star facility will get the Dorotha C. White Foundation certification as a flagship facility. A five star facility will get the DCW Foundation certification as an excellent facility. A four star rating will the certification as a good facility. Any facility under the four stars will not be allowed to participate in the "adopt a patient" program.

Why will the family of the patient agree to this? Studies have shown that visitation in nursing homes is at an all-time low due to odors, depressive surroundings, seeing the aging process as discouraging, observing the low esteem of the workers, insensitive providers, State and Federal enforcement tactics, etc. We believe that the "adopt a patient" program can bring positive forces to bear . . . volunteerism, benevolence, free services for cleaning and keeping the facility up, community services brought to the patient rather than vice versa. We believe the families are not visiting due to time restraints and families to raise, as well. So why not help them out and set an example that companionship makes a big difference in the patients will to live.

Why would the State and Federal regulators welcome this program? The goal of every surveyor I ever met was to improve the quality of life of those in nursing homes. Since it is not happening on a consistent basis and they know it, they will welcome it. And in fact many agencies are paying for most of these services in their Medicaid rate setting and not getting it. We all can see that the enforcement tactics do not work.

Why would a person in a community that has no loved one in a facility agree to do this? Why do we have people adopting foreign orphans, domestic foster children, keeping a highway clean, helping the elderly do their shopping, and helping the elderly stay warm or cool in inclement weather? Americans in fact do have a big heart when they know there is a need. In nursing homes the term Eldercide has been coined by the Foundation because the elderly are systematically institutionalized against their will and kept there until they die a lonely and scarred death. Elder Pride is the goal of the Foundation accomplished by adopting patients and eliciting outsiders to assist in the paradigm shift to a true quality of life on the inside.

www.dcwhitefoundation.org

Appendix V

PRESCRIPTION DRUG SIDE EFFECTS AND CHRONIC DISEASES

Chronic Diseases are the Leading Causes of Death and Disability in the U.S.

- 7 out of 10 deaths among Americans each year are from chronic diseases. Heart disease, cancer and stroke account for more than 50% of all deaths each year.
- In 2005, 133 million Americans—almost 1 out of every 2 adults—had at least one chronic illness.
- Obesity has become a major health concern. 1 in every 3 adults is obese3 and almost 1 in 5 youth between the ages of 6 and 19 is obese (BMI ≥ 95th percentile of the CDC growth chart).
- About one-fourth of people with chronic conditions have one or more daily activity limitations.
- Arthritis is the most common cause of disability, with nearly 19 million Americans reporting activity limitations.
- Diabetes continues to be the leading cause of kidney failure, non-traumatic lower-extremity amputations, and blindness among adults, aged 20-74.

- Excessive alcohol consumption is the third leading preventable cause of death in the U.S., behind diet and physical activity and tobacco.

Conventional Wisdom on the Four Common Causes of Chronic Disease

- Four modifiable health risk behaviors—lack of physical activity, poor nutrition, tobacco use, and excessive alcohol consumption—are responsible for much of the illness, suffering, and early death related to chronic diseases.
- More than one-third of all adults do not meet recommendations for aerobic physical activity based on the 2008 Physical Activity Guidelines for Americans, and 23% report no leisure-time physical activity at all in the preceding month.
- In 2007, less than 22% of high school students and only 24% of adults reported eating 5 or more servings of fruits and vegetables per day.
- More than 43 million American adults (approximately 1 in 5) smoke.
- In 2007, 20% of high school students in the United States were current cigarette smokers.
- Lung cancer is the leading cause of cancer death, and cigarette smoking causes almost all cases. Compared to nonsmokers, men who smoke are about 23 times more likely to develop lung cancer and women who smoke are about 13 times more likely. Smoking causes about 90% of lung cancer deaths in men and almost 80% in women. Smoking also causes cancer of the voice box (larynx), mouth and throat, esophagus, bladder, kidney, pancreas, cervix, and stomach, and causes acute myeloid leukemia.
- Excessive alcohol consumption contributes to over 54 different diseases and injuries, including cancer of the mouth, throat, esophagus, liver, colon, and breast,

liver diseases, and other cardiovascular, neurological, psychiatric, and gastrointestinal health problems.

- Binge drinking, the most dangerous pattern of drinking (defined as consuming more than 4 drinks on an occasion for women or 5 drinks for men) is reported by 17% of U.S. adults, averaging 8 drinks per binge.

- Side effects prescription drug use ranging from habit forming to death . . . the list in some cases is longer than the life it supposedly preserves . . . since prescription drugs do not rehabilitate but merely mask or provide temporary relief poly pharmacy (over medication) is a growing problem especially with the elderly. The advertisements promoting prescription drug use with the over whelming list of side effects should receive the same restrictions as alcohol and tobacco.

WHAT ABOUT THE USE OF PRESCRIPTION DRUGS AND A CORRELATION TO CHRONIC DISEASES AND LOSS OF IMMUNE RESISTANCE

Many of the more prevalent prescription drugs used by physician and patients to treat symptoms may have a correlation to causing chronic diseases and/or damaging the immune system. Chronic conditions such as heart disease, diabetes, COPD, CHF, respiratory failure, urinary failure, pancreatitis, liver disease, colon cancer, prostate cancer, appendicitis, CDIF, MERSA, stroke, lung disease, arthritis, etc. may be a result of the side effects of over medications and low immunity due to toxic chemical indulgence.

Diabetes

According to the CDC, an estimated 25.8 million (8.3 percent) Americans have diabetes. Of these, 7 million people are undiagnosed. Among those diagnosed, type 2 diabetes accounts for approximately 90 percent of all cases.

Jerry Rhoads

Diabetes is a leading cause of heart disease and stroke and is the seventh leading cause of death in the U.S. The exact causes of both type 1 and type 2 diabetes remain unknown; however, in the case of type 2, most risk factors are modifiable including: increased weight; physical inactivity; having high blood pressure; having abnormal cholesterol levels; and having high levels of triglycerides.

Depending on the type of diabetes, the treatment plan will differ; however, all will begin with lifestyle changes such as weight loss, physical activity, healthy diet and monitoring blood sugar levels.

A Good Immune System

"Our immune system is the most dynamic body component in determining our state of health or disease . . . Our immune system constantly interacts with our internal environment, protects us from our external environment and provides the inherent knowledge to sense the difference between friend and foe." Dr. Elson Haas

Dr. Bert Berkson, physician and researcher says, "Your immune system is constantly neutralizing the boundless toxins in our environment and fighting alien bacteria, fungi, protozoans and parasites. In addition, cancer cells are always appearing, and the immune system must be able to recognize and destroy them. A normal cell, in addition to destroying invaders, must remember who the invaders are, so that at a later date it can kill similar germs."

"The real threat comes from things like bacteria, viruses, fungi and parasites . . . those are the antigens (things that stimulate an immune response) that bring the immune system to a full state of alert." Dr. William Clark *At War Within*

The material including immune system disorders is offered to you for informational purposes only and is not meant to be interpreted as medical advice to diagnose, treat or cure any immune system disorder. You should consult with a qualified health professional whenever your health is in question.

PART II

Red Zone Thinking in Pursuit of The Self-Health End Zone

The following verse is quoted from Venice Bloodworth's wonderful book "The Key to Yourself". It puts the emphasis on thinking as being the way things materialize and turn into your dreams fulfilled. If we spend all of our energy wondering and worrying on how things will turn out we waste 85% of our time on this misspent energy and only use the 15% left to take actions based on our true beliefs hidden in our subconscious neural pathways. It is far more productive to stop worrying on things that don't occur 85% of the time and use this time to practice beliefs and take actions that will turn into your healthy, happy and prosperous life.

> *Finally, brethren whatsoever things are true, whatsoever things are honest, whatsoever things are just, whatsoever things are pure, whatsoever things are lovely and of good report; if there be any virtue and there be any praise, think on these things. The apostle Paul.*

"Most of us have overlooked the meaning of this verse. We have been so busy admiring its beauty of diction that we failed to place emphasis on the word think. If everybody followed Paul's injunction and thought only in terms of truth, honesty, justice, purity and loveliness, this world would be transformed from a planet of confusion, sickness and poverty into one of radiant health, happiness, and prosperity". Venice Bloodworth, psychologist

Jerry Rhoads

Quantum Physics is now the authentic basis for thoughts becoming things in our material world. Science has proven that we become what we think we are not why we are or who we are or when we will be our dream self. The Universe of energy and quantum particles that make up our material world are always changing to our mind's perception and commitment to self—actualization. If we feel that our life is controlled by a puppet string from heaven and we cannot control our destiny we have missed the opportunity to live in the vast continuum of our goals, dreams and hopes. I have learned through a study of the Science of self-health that self-determination is the formula and the mind's response to my soul's desires produces the results that we all want . . . a healthy, happy and prosperous life.

SELF-HEALTH DEFINED

You are the only one that can determine your life time . . . unless you get run over by a car . . . so the definition of Self-Health is the most important information you can receive:

S cience

E ngineered

L ife

F ulfillment

H ow you think determines your weight

E at when you are hungry and stop when you are full

A ge is not a factor to measure your longevity

L ife is your show and stage so act on it

T ime is a factor only in your use of it

H ealth is a journey not a destination

Healthy . . . Body . . . Mind . . . Heart . . . Soul = Self Health

Jerry Rhoads

A Self-Health Prescription

Pursuit of happiness is a process—think your way to

Desire
Dedication
Persistence
Thought
Effort
Work
Affirmation
Belief
Faith
Love
Health
Happiness
Prosperity

All of these are yours with the use of 365 days of verbal commitments to mind . . . body . . . heart . . . soul using your thoughts to change your mental and physical being to happy, healthy and prosperity.

In 1977, I didn't believe in myself let alone God and the power of belief. But I was forced to hang onto something. My job was gone, my career shattered, my aspirations in pieces before me. I turned to a discipline of thought that are still pulling me up to heights I've never known before. Just one year into depression I reworked my thoughts. The following poem says it best:

In the beginning I was born
In the end I will be reborn
Like a new sun
Each morn
Living each day hereafter
Giving hard work
With dedication and laughter

For I shall be free
To be what I want
To be
Free to create
Free to activate
The true pieces of happiness
365 times a year
Made peace by piece
With the past gone forever
Through each new endeavor
Cast with no regrets
Even as life shall cease
For the sun never sets
On a life in peace

I'm writing the thoughts I've had at the beginning of each day which carried me through *The Pursuit of the Health and Happiness End Zone*

I now believe in myself, in God, in the attainment of all my goals. I'm convinced anyone who can conceive a thought in which they believe, shall believe in themselves, in God (the personification of belief) and shall achieve their own form of success. For, success is the attainment of what a person can conceive and believe in until it becomes a reality. It's the attainment of peace; peace in knowing you're whole, not pieces.

I believe you can find the same peace by reading my *daily sayings, affirmations and confirmations (which I used as prayers), to build for the first time your self-image, self-worth, self-capital, self-confidence, self-health and your belief in values which can't fail.*

Kindness
Giving
Loving

189

This is the Pursuit of Health and Happiness

WILL, WILLING AND WILLED
BY: JERRY RHOADS

I CAN, I WILL, I AM
TO MAKE IT HAPPEN
I CAN SEE THE VISION
I WILL UNDERSTAND
BEING IS WILLING
IT TO HAPPEN
IN THE FUTURE
BY INSTILLING
THE HABIT
THE EFFORT
THE ROUTINE
TO DO IT
NO AMOUNT OF FEAR
CAN OVERCOME
MY WILL
TO ENDURE
FOR I HAVE BEEN WILLED
THE RIGHT
TO BE
AS FEAR IS KILLED
BY MY THINKING
AND MY FAITH
TO BE MORE THAN
DOUBT AS MY BEING

Values

What is valuable to you? Remarkably, the answer to this question will have a great deal to do with determining your destiny. Whereas attitudes of mind are important to the striving for goals and seeking of goals, attitudes are dependent upon the value structure of an individual. The proposition "Which comes first, values or attitudes?" can be compared to the question "What comes first, the brick or the mortar?" Obviously, we always need both to be able to build a strong, unyielding structure.

Therefore, both values and attitudes are needed to construct a character. The values are the bricks and the mortar is the attitudes. The word value is the base of the word "valuable". Values are also the base of a valuable character. To better understand this, I would like to discuss values. I should specify these are my values now; but it is my feeling to be able to grow as an individual, values have to grow and change.

The attitude to expand values is the stabilizer to the character we all are trying to build. My primary values are: self-acceptance through the establishment of worthwhile goals and striving to attain them; self-expression through the interaction with all kinds of people and the education of my family; self-respect through the appreciation of the accomplishments of others; self-confidence through satisfaction of worthwhile accomplishments; self-development through striving for new ideas and new ways of doing things.

(I think it is important to note in this summary there is no mention of money as a self—value. It really becomes a result of applying values. It is the measuring stick of the progress being made in implementing values in everyday life.)

Values must be constructed by a set of attitudes in fitting together peace. Values are important in work. Values are important in social life. Values are important in maintaining physical vitality. Values are important in constructing the spiritual side of your life.

Work	Social
Body	Spirit

"House of Happiness"

The values of work.

To me, the value to achieve results through helping others is the fulcrum for work values. The art of helping others is not easy to come by. It takes a certain amount of self-sacrifice. But in the process, it eliminates threat and builds rapport. The helpful attitude is a positive attitude. It is basically unselfish. It helps one to see the other person's point of view. It creates a very good environment for cooperation and communication. How can anyone refuse help and how could anyone that is offering to help not gain the other person's attention. Another important value of work is competence. To strive for knowledge, in your endeavors, must pay off. This desire can only result in better skills. Better skills result in better results. Competence can only come from a systematic and habitual study program. Self-development is a continuing every day process. It's like good physical conditioning, it takes self-discipline. It takes tolerance to discomfort and pain, and it takes the desire to improve. For the successful person, it is a habit attained. For the struggling person, it is passing thought.

Another value of work is teaching others the competence you've attained. In teaching others, you learn more yourself. In teaching others, you develop a sense of teamwork and cooperation. Again, it establishes the lines of communication on an unthreatened basis. Teaching is satisfying. Teaching is as natural as learning. All the teacher has to do is have the desire to pass on the knowledge to others. How can we have learning without teaching? Teaching requires the ability to communicate, verbally and in writing. It stimulates the mind to think in broader and deeper terms. It stimulates ideas because it requires the capability to attract the attention of the student, retain attention and evaluate the results of the efforts.

Another value of work is challenge. Challenge is the food for achievement. Achievement is the food for enthusiasm and effort. Enthusiasm and effort are the food for success. Success is not a result. It is a means to happiness. Talent is either imposed by or developed by the mind. The situation normally is secondary because it is merely environmental and normally does not impose limitations on the success as much as the way the mind conceives the challenge. So it depends upon the manner in which the mind conceives the endeavor and the degree of challenge it represents. The more stimulated and disciplined the mind, the higher the degree of the challenge, and in many cases, the higher the degree of stimulation.

You take away the challenge and you take away the incentive to strive. Efforts become unworthy. Achievement is shallow.

Once conquered, the challenge becomes history. And the next step is the future in yet another more demanding and stimulating experience. Challenge has a great impact on the amount of work a person will delegate to others. If the mind isn't stimulated by the need of stronger and stronger challenges, the mind will not look to others for help, but will continue to do work which won't result in fulfilled accomplishment. The mind stimulated by challenge must go on to more demanding situations and in doing so, will delegate the less challenging projects to others. With this infallible logic, you will find that to motivate people and to delegate, you must continually challenge your own abilities first, then make sure there are rewards lucrative enough to establish an incentive for others to attain and meet the same degree of challenge.

Another value of work is recognition. Recognition is a personality need. It is the result of needing other people. To admit you need other people is to admit you need to give before you attain recognition. Recognition for the sake of recognition is not possible. Other people will not give it unless they feel it is earned sincerely. I feel it's not what you think you are worth that counts, it counts more if you prove to others what you're worth. This is the route to obtaining recognition. One cannot expect results without first getting results. To get results requires putting the emphasis upon the act of giving and not upon recognition as the purpose. Recognition should not be subjective, nor the objective. If it's detected by others you're striving only to get acceptance from them, and they will be less likely to give it. If you're able to put recognition into perspective as the result of worthwhile goals, the attainment will come much easier. The attainment of recognition is a result and not the means, or the reason for the act.

Another value of work is immortality. The building of a legend is every man's dream. Building a legend is a successful man's epitaph. Since the results are dependent upon the individual, it's how the individual acts that determines his impact on the world. To work for results is to work for the legend. To work for work's sake is to accept mediocrity. Those that don't accept mediocrity will somehow leave their mark on eternity. To look back upon the great men in our history is to look back upon ordinary human beings striving for a purpose. Therefore, to have a purpose is to strive for immortality. Why should we want immortality? Why did Edison want electricity? Why did Alexander Graham Bell want the telephone? Why did the Wright Brothers want to fly? Why did Henry Ford want an automobile? It was much more than monetary rewards that they were seeking. They were looking for etchings in their fellow man's memories; and they got it. The only way to get immortality is to want it so badly that it becomes a purpose so overwhelming, it must come to pass.

The Values of a social life.

Ironically, the values of your social life aren't much different than values of work. There is the desire to be accepted. You will note I said accepted, not necessarily liked. The social system is a means of balancing our values. Without the balance we wouldn't have laws; we wouldn't have rationality in our lives. We would have nothing to govern nor establish guideposts for a way of life. Acceptance then is conformity to social law. To practice good work values will lead to worthy social values. For the worthy, tenor of work carries through a soothing tone for all of life.

The values of physical well-being.

It is amazing that the well-developed value system and attitude of mind carries through to a concern for physical well-being. Most people healthy mentally, are also healthy physically. The desire to maintain oneself mentally carries through to the body. Physical well-being is a release of mental frustration. It allows the body to throw off tension and nervous anxiety. Physical fitness or mental fitness go hand in hand. To look at the embodiment of success is to dissect a healthy body. If a body isn't resilient, it is difficult to imagine it having the energy, the drive and determination it takes to have a healthy mind. Interestingly, I see a correlation between the man who likes to compete and stay physically healthy, and the man who likes to compete in life and stay mentally healthy. The person who avoids physical competition and challenge more than likely will avoid responsibility, authority, and the challenge of business.

In physical fitness, the concern should be more for the results you're trying to attain than the means you use. Many endeavors are status symbols which really don't provide a healthy frame of mind or body. Because there must be enjoyment. Without the capability of attaining some feeling of release and achievement, it's hard to imagine the activity will be worthwhile. Look at children. It's just as important for them to be educated physically as it is to be educated mentally.

Unfortunately, our society isn't giving as much priority to physical well-being as it should. We do have an emphasis on athletics, which is good. It trains the body as well as the mind. The physically fit person will also be able to function at a higher energy level and is likely to have a fuller sexual life. Sexuality has a great dependence on the body's physical well-being. The healthier the body, the healthier the sex experience. All are ingredients to a full life.

The values of the spiritual life.

Organized religion is not necessarily the media for constructing the spiritual element of a person. Spiritual vitality may merely be a state of mind. The desires and needs and purposes of the other values may be a result of having a healthy, spiritual state of mind. They speak of the Bible as being The Good Book. To this I agree. It is one of many Good Books. All books relating to the positive elements of our well-being are good books. Any book which proposes a better mode of conduct, a better mode of activity, and a better mode of living should be called a good book.

Anything constructive which develops the state of mind should be called spiritual. Therefore, it is possible the positive state of mind is a form of spiritual fulfillment. Believing positively, you're doing the right thing, is likely an act of the spiritual. Love for others must also be an element of the spiritual. The desire to improve oneself and others also must be a part of it. This leads one to believe there can be heaven on earth, once the state of mind is such that acceptance and help to others is of first importance. To really enjoy helping others is to be fulfilled. This is the attainment of the spiritual.

Many organized religions require that the participant be dependent upon a mode of conduct to attain spiritual fulfillment. It almost becomes an addiction. It's hard to believe this is the most productive form of spiritual activity. The intent of many of the religions is to attain a state of mind which will allow a person to conduct themselves in a positive worthwhile manner; however, in their enactment they compel the participant to submit to a ritual which is neither understood nor believed. Then, for the sake of attaining the spiritual at the time of death, they must conform to the ritual. On the other hand, an emphasis on the spiritual in the development of a positive value system, exercised by a positive attitude seems to be more productive.

This puts the emphasis on the enactment of a good value system now, for the purpose of attaining happiness now, and not just a submission to a process that allows for attainment of heaven later; while heaven on earth is readily attainable. Why not develop the state of mind, as the attainment of the spiritual, rather than submission to dogmatic rules. The positive puts the emphasis upon the attainment of a healthy state of mind, and not on the negative fear of not attaining the spiritual fulfillment, if you break the rules. Mental development puts the action in the mind of the person, rather than submission to the soothsayers.

Unfortunately, most denominations of Christianity require a conformity to a commitment so one can believe in a process. In other words, you must believe in a process so you can attain eternal happiness after death. Happiness for the living doesn't carry a high priority. This is done without an attempt to define God. To define God as being a good healthy spiritual state of mind is so simple, it is attractive to the pragmatist. To believe in a healthy state of mind, is to believe in God. There is no need to be concerned about the later existence of heaven or hell for heaven and hell exist on earth today, tomorrow, and in the future. Mortals create their own heaven or hell, and the attainment of one or the other depends on the state of mind. Happiness is in the mind of the living, and the attainment of eternal life must be left to a process not to be understood.

The primer for a healthy state of mind is the teachings of the Bible, the Ten Commandments and the book of love. The "Good Books" have established the framework for teachings which enable the students to formulate a proper state of mind. Those that learn this can't fail to be healthy spiritually. Happiness is to recognize positive thoughts are a worthwhile need and a worthwhile value, and must be attained. The person who does this is spiritually healthy.

The person who doesn't do this is spiritually unhealthy and more than likely living in hell here on earth. This is the way it should be. This is life itself. How can we deny the laws of nature which are the closest we'll get to finding the supernatural, until we die. Ultimately, the laws of nature and man emanate from the law of cause and effect. The amount of effort, sincerity, quality, you put into the cause will determine the effect. Therefore the amount of sincerity, effort, and quality you put into the pursuit of a healthy, spiritual state of the subconscious mind will determine the happiness you will get in your conscious lifetime.

From the Red Zone to the Self-Health living everyday

We all have values within the framework of attitudes, holding the pieces of life together. Hopefully yours are healthy. If not, try my prescription for happiness. It has taken most successful, fulfilled people years of unhappiness and trial and error to discover the worthwhile benefits of positive mental processes. Their philosophy is at the point where they retrain their subconscious mind to attain worthwhile goals, and implement what the conscious mind is conceiving as worthwhile goals, so they are able to help and influence other people. They will also leave the world a little better place. This is true happiness. For the attainment of a positive, healthy subconscious mind is what creates heavenly peace and happiness here on earth.

In the attached daily exercises we must reprogram the subconscious mind from a failure mode to a success mode. But first we need to understand that failure is a perception not a permanent location in the brain. To brain wash the negative and input the positive into the subconscious mind will take some time. For me it took a year of writing down positive thoughts. After the year became history my conscious mind was set on achieving and believing not deceiving my subconscious self-worth. Try it . . . It works.

"Failure is a figment of human imagination
Dwelling on the negative makes it happen
Given time even a monkey can fail"

Are you ever sure you're a failure or
Is it just your mother's opinion that becomes yours or
Was it your or her impression of your Father

We all have fears that come from dreams reposes
Time tells us it is too late and we believe it
Even though others have been awarded the roses

However, life is not a destination but a journey
Meant to be at your direction and fortune
Whether rich or poor, in sickness or health

The avoidance of failure is not wealth
But only a fleeting surge of pride that subsides
And leaves the dreamer in for a nightmare

So this book is not about failure but success
Daily thoughts that propel us forward
Into tomorrow in spite of doubt and fear of the unknown

I call it the "Prescription for Health and Happiness"
Because it takes the mind off of the expectation of failure
And put the words of success into our subconscious brain power

Forging a habit and thought process inseparable
And tied to perpetual faith not needing a God to save us
But a belief in self as the savior

Take this trip with me and you shall never fear
The action and will benefit from the act
Until you have an addiction for the love of life

For if you love you can be loved
If you are loved you are connected to eternity
And its mighty pull towards fulfillment . . . By the
Universal Spirit and its Law of Attraction

When I started my own business my daughter Kim said I needed to make sure I stayed healthy because who would pay the bills if I got sick. She even advised me on how to stay healthy . . . jump rope . . . so I did . . . but I still felt sick when I contemplated the loneliness of a new venture with no means of support. So I also needed to keep my mind in shape so I wrote a thought each day for the first 365 days so I could sustain my positive attitude towards the future by repeating and rereading what I had written each day for my vision of the future.

This is my story in positive affirmations (prayers) using poetry as the median to retrain my subconscious mind for conceiving and achieving what I am believing:

Poetry is for those senses
That need expression
To knock down fences
Concealing creation

Day One

You have given me a day
I will give you back in every way
For my time well spent
Leads to the advent

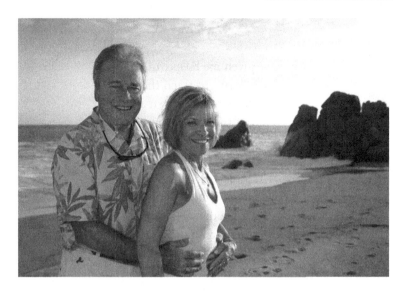

Day Two

You have provided me desire
To direct others towards acts that inspire
And blessings never to expire

Day Three

You have given me health
I feel the need to spread myself
With wings of abundant wealth

Day Four

Sunshine and Cloudy skies are your signs
I want to fly between those lines
Understanding the verses and the rhymes

Jerry Rhoads

Day Five

You have given me beautiful children
I will strive to teach them
To be the good as heaven above
And the face of love

Day Six

Give me guidance in my work
Be it good; so be it not
I will be more than an ordinary ink spot

Day Seven

Good blessings for all I know
May be enemy or foe
Telling me to grow

Day Eight

God lead me to the light
I will not partake
Until the time is right
And the fruit is ripe

Day Nine

Help me be patient and understanding
For in righteousness comes a soft landing
On a hard runway

Day Ten

I must know my goals to seek a destiny . . .
For the journey is not free,
In the country of "tis of thee"

Day Eleven

Light my way with wise markings
If I lose my way,
Shed your light on my shadow
Before it goes away

Day Twelve

Up with truth . . . idolize it
If it can't be said
Say nothing . . . don't disguise it

Day Thirteen

Blessed be thy ways
Help me find them
By loving the "J" word
In the hymn showing the way

Day Fourteen

How can today be more?
Make it so . . .
With more dedication;
To cultivate the deed you sow

Day Fifteen

Fly with me to the moon
Thrill us all
Adventure isn't over by noon
Nor does the star dim at night fall

Day Sixteen

Help them who help me
If they do,
How can anyone best us?

Day Seventeen

Hail to those who restrain
For they are never vain
And win the final frame

Day Eighteen

Faith is a figment with a smile
Without it,
Is to struggle each and every mile

Day Nineteen

Find me a wind to ride
And I will give you a bottle in the tide
With a message of hopes and pride

Day Twenty

Look for more and find less;
Look for less and find more
Look and you shall find no profit
In gaining the apple and losing the core

Day Twenty-one

Don't commit thyself to wrath
Tis not the right path . . .
Nor does it hath
The sheep before the staff

Day Twenty-two

Find a shepherd to herd them
Let it be me
For I will love them, stern to stem

Day Twenty-three

Temptation is not an enemy
Tis human;
But it will not control thee;
For that enemy is me

Day Twenty-four

Bygone are the insecure moments
For yet the happier remembrance
Will emerge from more mature wits

Day Twenty-five

Finding ways to do good is easy
The strength to do good
If you are scant and breezy
Is rather tense and queasy

Day Twenty-six

Award me a way of believing
Help those who are deceiving
me for believing
To be just like me

Day Twenty-seven

Not believing is painful . . . relieve the pain
By deceiving the source of pain
With bad seeds planted as good deeds

Day Twenty-eight

Forgotten are the tender words
Revive and relive them to be yours
At any age and on every page

Day Twenty-nine

Days pass as grains of time
Savor the eternal sand pile
As your past and future
Become your now

Day Thirty

Pity those who are shallow
For their field of dreams is forever fallow
Of sincerity, health and prosperity

Day Thirty-one

Reality Does Not Make Us
We Make Reality

Day Thirty-two

Salute those who struggle to win
Their will shan't be throttled,
But by doubt from within

Day Thirty-three

Forgive those who spite
They will live their lesson;
Never learning what's right

Day Thirty-four

Never give up . . . never fear it . . . so be it
That right is won and wrong is done,
For the will to be righteous is the living spirit

Day Thirty-five

Lose with grace and try again
Loyalty to one's purpose
And principles will ever win

Day Thirty-six

Praise those who know the secret
For they shall beget the truth
About the onset of eternal wisdom

Day Thirty-seven

A mind up for a challenge
Has energy and vantage . . .
And the intelligence to engage hope

Day Thirty-eight

Challenge, like good music shall never age
If it is the right vintage
And the right stage

Day Thirty-nine

I get the message
From the postman in a bottle . . .
Unless I'm an addict to myself
Looking for the throttle

Day Forty

Will and desire to persist,
Like money in the bank
Rewards the withdrawal of
Ill will to cease and desist

Day Forty-one

Holiness is not necessarily happiness
But without it,
One may become Cane or Able

Day Forty-two

Silence is awaiting space
To listen is to create a place
For the silence to be heard
In a miracle or its lasting word

Day Forty-three

Together we thrive . . .
Like sun and weeds
Separated we're scant alive . . .
In work and deeds

Day Forty-four

Determined to be, am I
Something forever, that will not die . . .
Like the free bird in a deep blue sky

Day Forty-five

Trust is a song;
Sing it and you will find the call
Deceit doesn't sing;
Sling it and you will hit the wall

Day Forty-six

Express your feelings
By pen and act
Reveal your thoughts
To those masses who react

Day Forty-seven

Day into darkness gone
With no purpose is light
But the darkness shedding truth
Is to shine beyond a sunless night

Day Forty-eight

Lead those who must follow,
Be the righteous man, do not fail
For they who blindly follow
Are not the wise men nor the Holy Grail

Day Forty-nine

We live, we give, we are
More than twinkles of a distant star . . .
Less than our dreams afar
And our past by far

Day Fifty

To quit is to be close To the one
Who knows all and does little
And is the demise of the rainbow
Forsaken with no place to go

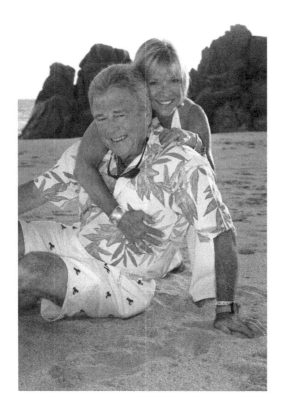

Day Fifty-one

Gone are the yesterdays; say goodbye
Savor today; for it too must die tomorrow
And you will have the last say

Day Fifty-two

Sunshine is made by a better mood
Shunning thought not to brood . . .
Not to doubt not to have an attitude

Day Fifty-three

Put off the schemes that might have been
To another day
Then pursue your dreams
And visualize another way

Day Fifty-four

Gather the flock, pray for peace
Quiet the flock, comb their fleece;
For hope will never cease

Day Fifty-five

Earth is heaven for the winners
Hell is here on earth for the sinners
As sure as bad blood simmers
And muscle trimmers

Day Fifty-six

Forget not why you're here
Remember you should not fear
For there is no fright
In actions made right

Day Fifty-seven

Search your mind for the answers
Teach the questions
To the searchers of truth . . .
Then learn from them

Day Fifty-eight

Create a friend and you have
Some time to spend
Create an enemy and you have
Nothing but an ex friend

Day Fifty-nine

Faith, hope and charity
Heals the mind and
A healthy mind
Doesn't leave the body far behind

Day Sixty

Make the trip that you've cast
Pick your banner and wave its mast;
Let it flap . . . then pledge yourself to a better map

Day Sixty-one

Sixty stanzas have emanated
None would have come to pass
If I had procrastinated
About being first not last

Day Sixty-two

Without reality,
A passing would seem like an illusion
But for me life is living so you feel
Your elusive dream until it is real

Sixty-three

Forgotten are the reasons why
Men either do or don't before they die
Then the epitaph is but a lie

Day Sixty-four

Aaron, Rebecca, Job and John
Made their way from Babylon
So we could find our way to the Kingdom

Day Sixty-five

"Heretic, rebel the dirty lout
Drew a circle to shut me out
Love and I had the wit to win
We drew a "bigger" circle and took him in"
Markham and Rhoads

Day Sixty-six

Fathers and sons write the song
Mothers and daughters sing along
Husbands and wives beget the song
Sisters and Brothers must get along

Day Sixty-seven

Gallant stand the law of immortal men
Shredded, it will withstand
The legions of mortal sin
As an epitaph to the moral man

Day Sixty-eight

Do we know nature's secret yet
Even though we see the sun set
And the rain wet
Still beyond the Internet

Day Sixty-nine

Heathens alert us to your cause
Our efforts must act to mend the flaws;
Now, without pause
Restore a belief in Santa Claus

Day Seventy

To stop thinking is unthinkable
To think of stopping is unstoppable
For those who are thoughtful
The mind never sleeps

Day Seventy-one

Our calling is just forming,
Listen up boys;
For we are babes in a wilderness of noise
And lost toys

Day Seventy-two

Beauty and understanding
Is in our hearts
The object is to find where it starts
And how it mends our hurts

Day Seventy-three

Vital principles cannot waiver
In the wind of doubt
Strive to save them before you savor,
Their immense clout

Day Seventy-four

For those who don't love themselves
Find out that they pay
The price of twelve's . . .
Six times two little love each day

Day Seventy-five

Align yourself with those who can
and do
Avoid those with attitudes of
Don't, Can't, Won't, thrown at you

Day Seventy-six

Our children frame the picture of what we are
Look at them to find,
If you're a dark shadow
Or shining star

Day Seventy-seven

The morning mist and evening prayer
Will cleanse
Each fortnight
You spend with friends

Day Seventy-eight

A smile reflects more than warmth
It opens your book of character
And allows the reader to find faith
In the life your write

Day Seventy-nine

Hello sweet reality, goodbye insecurity
A change is coming over me . . .
Can't you see
I am now free to be me

Day Eighty

Winning isn't everything
But the will to win is
So long as the fight is
Right

Day Eighty-one

Life is an exciting journey
For those who travel it every day,
To find their way and
Expect to get it back as combat pay

Day Eighty-two

Control your mind
And you can control self
Control your principles
And others will follow in sickness and in health

Day Eighty-three

Fighting against wrong doing is a creed
Turning your back
On a friend is undoing for greed

Day Eighty-four

Look around for disciples against sin
They're waiting in ever moving circles . . .
Take them in

Day Eighty-five

Give me this day for service
To man kind
And I will do my best
To serve those left behind

Day Eighty-six

Live for love and you'll find it
For a life without love is lost,
And those who fear love
Will not go near it

Day Eighty-seven

Honor your principles before the Judge
For the Judge stands on your honor
To not worship judgmental minds

Day Eighty-eight

Find someone to lead to better
Or fall in behind
And follow the trend setter

Day Eighty-nine

Slamming the door on a friend
Is like spitting into the wind;
A fatal regret to get all wet

Day Ninety

Fight yourself and lose
Love yourself,
To fight the blues

Day Ninety-one

A gull in flight is beauty
To light on earth is necessity, not duty . . .
So praise the sky
And wonder why we can't fly

Day Ninety-two

Find a way to the chemical sojourn
And as your cares burn into a habitual down turn
Give it up and throw off the urge to purge fear

Day Ninety-three

Silence isn't sound to the deaf
As a mountain isn't without a cliff
And a forest green without a leaf . . . it is what it is

Day Ninety-four

Take only what is needed
As self-indulgence has been exceeded
Till morals and moderation must be heeded

Day Ninety-five

Upbringing and character,
What's it to ya
Everything, hallelujah

Day Ninety-six

Utter shallow phrases
And you will receive fallow praises
As the boom-a-rang effect raises
It's eventual return to waste us

Day Ninety-seven

Alert yourself to pick up a banner
For with no purpose,
Is a losing manner
Likely to surface

Day Ninety-eight

Pick up the pen and express
For silence is unrest
"Words scorned, digest
Those being left at rest"

Day Ninety-nine

Foster no ill will unto me
For I will not dare fight thee . . .
Unless I'm not free
To fight for my country

Day One Hundred

Sunrise is for seeing the hope in another day
If you don't open your eyes to the skies,
A frown can delay Life's size
While a smile is Life's prize

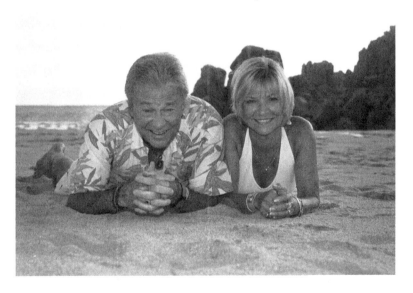

Day 101

Grieve no longer child
Of no one
Your Mother is not beguiled . . .
She is gone . . . Make her memory your child

Day 102

Hasten my friend,
Know thyself
Then hasten to teach your friend
External happiness and Internal health

Day 103

The smitten heart
Is sensitive to other times
A sensitive heart writes
About poetic times, lines and rhymes

Day 104

Seek not friend or foe
Instead look for peace
To know
the difference
And praise its existence

Day 105

The bible draws good signs
Many hidden between
The bad times
And forgone lines

Day 106

My heart cries out ideals
And my ears are closed to deals
While my head says I might
If this is wrong; what is right

Day 107

How, I cry; why can't I
Get through to show the why
And wherefore we must die
Or is eternity just a lie

Day 108

Don't let yourself believe in less
For there is always
More belief in happiness
And less in unhealthy stress

Day 109

Up with your eyes to find
What may be night and day
As the dust of decay
Will cloud your vision,
Any other way

Day 110

There's more for the knowing soul
By knowing thyself,
By knowing thy goal
. . . a prayer of knowing, a willful foal

Day 111

Afterwards, what can I say
Just words held over from yesterday
And re-spoken today
As Affirmation without display

Day 112

Damn; I cry, I am!
Listen world; I sigh, I can!
Whatever the bill, I will it seems!
Then reality catches up with my dreams.

Day 113

Kiss the hand and you will eternally receive
Bite the hand and you'll always grieve
Shake the hand and
Even the will of God won't deceive

Day 114

I talk but does it matter?
Are the ears just hearing chatter?
Does it scatter above the clatter?
Sure it does . . . for I believe in the father, son
and heaven's ladder.

Day 115

Guide my eyes to better places
Turned into contented faces
and holy Graces
Opening the door to play Kings and Aces

Day 116

Born to be free
With nothing better to be . . .
Then as a moving part of a family tree
Growing inside of me

Day 117

Can help be had
For those who pause
As the lion and scare crows
Turned bad
In the land of OZ

Day 118

When I get through
To the promise land
Will ears be listening
and eyes glistening
So I can see and understand?

Day 119

Cry out and you will be heard
For the still are quieting the herd . . .
Taught minding the immortal word
By ignoring the lies and the absurd

Day 120

Tired or content; who can tell?
But those held by pleasure
Will certainly dwell
on lost treasure

Day 121

Where do the peace doves flock
I would welcome them
To my warlock dock
Where the flock's fleece
Is shorn for the deceased

Day 122

Helping others to become
Is smart not dumb . . . even for the lowly sum
Of two plus two, fortunes are won

Day 123

Foster principles in your softer mind
To gain the gift of being not unkind . . .
and ye shall find a way to being that kind

Day 124

Honor is for those who earn it
and are honorable;
To ask for the pride of honor
Without earning it is dishonorable

Day 125

Greatness is not reserved for Kings and Queens
It's waiting for minds
With Roots and Wings
And a Heart that sings

Day 126

Before your life's puzzle can be solved
The pieces must be a shove
So the edges are all involved
As the first and last piece is love
With relationships fully evolved . . .

Day 127

Throw off the mental chains
Release your potential gains
For earning self-worth has its pains

Day 128

Thank God the storms aren't in tune
And we can't cut down the moon
For it is much too soon
To ride around the world in a Hot Air Balloon

Day 129

What a man thinks he will become,
Becomes what he is and what he denies,
Becomes what he thinks isn't
Leftover or pleasant

Day 130

Old age may not be so much wise or couth
As it proves what is unfound by youth . . .
An acceptance of just living
For what life is giving . . . then paying it back.

Day 131

Tell me something, I can grind
Into grain, for a hungry mind
Then take it and make it into fine
Wine for those left behind

Day 132

My Children, all four
How can parenthood be much more
You are the core for evermore
And what's in store

Day 133

Children of innocence
Is it lost to adolescence
Or is it the guilt of mankind
Leading us from behind

Day 134

Creation of a life's attitude
Determines an epitaph's
Magnitude and altitude

Day 135

Nowhere do we find in writing
Daily thoughts that are exciting
Unless we look in this book
Or find it in your Nook

Day 136

Yesterday echoes across
The canyon of knowledge
But knowledge only hears
The sound of tomorrow's adage

Day 137

Pelted with nonsensical noise
A world needs a voice with sensual poise
Passionate prose and hearty toys
For life boils down to girls and boys

Day 138

Beauty is a face in love
Regardless of the stars above
The look of love is a beautiful place
Here or in love's inner space

Day 139

Silence is the music of lovers
Make the music from silence
By giving passion for
The doubt under the covers

Day 140

Who are we to say who will be chosen
on Judgment Day
It could be anyone, anywhere for any reason
if they pray . . . Amen

Day 141

Forgotten are the meek
Looking to find
What they seek . . . [peace and quiet]
Below the radar and above the riot

Day 142

Foolish is the man who fails to
Learn from lessons in his wake
That Washes away his failures
Leaving everything at stake

Day 143

Creation is in the eyes of the artist
Let them see before they create
The eyes of mortals
Depicting life and fate

Day 144

Life and death is not the beginning nor the end
It's merely a starting and stopping point to another time
So wind up your watch and watch the time fly by
And believe that the soul will never die

Day 145

Growing older is exciting
So long as life's inviting
And inciting . . .
More each day
With less decay

Day 146

People are straight or tipped
Acting roles without a script
Saying things they don't mean
Wanting to be the center of the scene
Waiting for God's sin fighter to redeem

Day 147

Faith is Hope conceived
Created by a God perceived
As the Maker of men
Leaving fear deceived
and souls relieved of sin

Day 148

Hurry after happiness
It is so hard to catch unless
You are into being helpless
Then it is useless

Day 149

Fight against those who neglect and abuse
Right says they are bound to lose
Left to their devices and vices to choose

Day 150

Flock behind the true leader's whip
The followers flock for leadership
And seek to find fulfillment
In faith not dissent

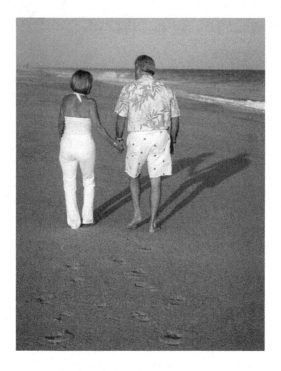

Day 151

Creation of a lasting thought
Is more than one that is impulsively bought
Or a dropped ball thought caught

Day 152

Focus your mind on others
Embrace yourself and your brothers
Given Time, Space and Druthers

Day 153

Accepting others for what they are
Will bring you up
And take you far

Day 154

Awareness of the finite being
Takes depth of insight unseeing
With belief that we are connected
Yet fleeing our very being

Day 155

Philosophy of life comes
From thought
Not just inherited life
Or material bought

Day 156

Fallacies come from weaker minds
Not Einstein's
While a strength of doubt confines
A simpler mind to matter [E=MC2]

Day 157

Beautiful cornfields are the picture perfect
Invisible to the city
And its scripture
Stated for convenience not nature

Day 158

The female creature
Beloved is magic
But not loved she is tragic
Waiting for another feature

Day 159

Something for nothing is nonsense
As is trading a pound for a sixpence
Everything made by common sense
Is making a dollar out of risk's suspense

Day 160

Blessed with a heart and soul
The skin covers us all,
But some aren't to be as whole
If their mind lags behind
The sign of the times

Day 161

Godliness is human heredity
Passed by genes filled with uncertainty
Thought restored by the divinity
Hidden somewhere amongst infinity

Day 162

Stubbornness will narrow the mind
Those that narrow themselves,
Never will find their mind
Nor both sides of their behind

Day 163

Truth is an invention of humans
To answer questions
And to explain omens
Yet to be true blue missions

Day 164

Sadness is to realize weakness
Brought on by selfishness
Void of tenderness
Justified by stubbornness

Day 165

Grateful are the givers
For they too shall receive
Of themselves
For themselves
By themselves

Day 166

Hail those who think they can
For no challenge is too hard to span
Including the globe and Uncle Sam

Day 167

Enthusiasm is the fire
To qualify us
For hire and does not require
Something that will expire

Day 168

Goodliness is a trait hard earned
Contrary to hate that's easily spurned
Godliness is a faith well earned
Contrary to doubt that's easily discerned

Day 169

Beauty is in your mind
Especially if you're so inclined,
to look forward not behind

Day 170

Spite is a futile trait
That separates love and hate
Into fate

Day 171

Marvel at the strongest
They may start out as the weakest
Only to become strong, then best
By overtaking those at rest

Day 172

Supreme beings are here it seems
Amongst us—
Touch them as they pass
By your dreams and schemes
Into the past

Day 173

March to your own drum beat,
But honor the drummer's feat
That moves your conceit
Away from lies and deceit

Day 174

The body needs a soul
To warm the heart and guide
The spirit towards its goal
And hang on for the bumpy ride

Day 175

Utterances of love
Come from within; speak back
And forever be at peace
With your mate and love's pact

Day 176

Take me into your trust
I will support you—taunted or cussed
Fear as you might, curse as you must
The memory bank will never go bust

Day 177

The psalm of life is sensitivity
Expressed in words of creativity
Formed by acts that will last in infamy
Unless selfishness is the epitome
Of that life.

Day 178

Thinking of another time
Is putting timeless thoughts
Into a rhyme
Above the thwarts of crime
Or the threats of the Devine

Day 179

Don't we humans behold the sky
Mountains only help for they never die
While animals walk and fly
Holding onto evolution as they decay and die

Day 180

The day in the life of a nobody,
If dedicated to somebody,
Will be remembered by everybody

Day 181

Thoughts can seek the deepest meaning
If plotted towards others called brothers
Be they uplifting not demeaning

Day 182

Cradle to grave, most don't know
What direction they must go . . . so take a chance
Give your love for romance
And life will fill your cradle
And honor your grave for circumstance

Day 183

Praise the days
For the darkest nights
Shall soon be the dawn
Of better ways

Day 184

Alas, clouds are fleeting,
Don't close their eyes
To this illusion's demise
They merely pass under unknown skies
Floating in and out of our brain's mortal size

Day 185

A Guitar and a boy play's a tune
Practiced in his room
Taking us around the moon
Waiting for a piano and a bassoon
To combat his Father's gloom

Day 186

Patience is blue, temper is red
Blend the two
And you have bled blue blood
That is ready for peace held true

Day 187

Chemical talent from uppers and downers,
Pills and thrills, has few skills
And self-destruction is what fear distills
So replace those refills with what belief wills

Day 188

Wake up . . . subconscious mind for your own sake
With peace, love, health, happiness and prosperity
Otherwise your body of work is destined
For an early wake

Day 189

Live life without fear
As positive thoughts are near
Then ask and ye shall believe
That life is better given to receive
Than lost to deceive

Day 190

Surely you don't expect miracles
When all you are looking for
Are more immovable obstacles

Day 191

My head rocks of ages
My eyes roll with Bible pages
But my life is fulfilled by Sex, Kids and Rock & Roll
As the depth of happiness and baring my soul

Day 192

Natural highs are speed to freedom
Unnatural highs are speed to oblivion
"Uncontrolled speed to get high" is a risky idiom
For an empty stadium

Day 193

Silence is purity, don't fade it
Speak and you close your ears
And only hear your own fears
With no plans to avoid being afraid

Day 194

For those who believe in the will; will find the way!
Their day will come, their night has been,
Tomorrow is hope from within

Day 195

Thoughts continued for today
Bring thoughts of no sorrow
For today's happiness is for those
That live today as if there's no tomorrow

Day 196

Pilots of the earth
Guide us from infant birth
Into ourselves beyond our mortal girth

Day 197

Know thyself
And thyself will know happiness
Reject your self
And the self will die of loneliness

Day 198

Accept thyself
So others can accept themselves
For your sake
And quell their habit to forsake you and them

Day 199

Take no gifts
Before giving
Make no enemies
Before living
He who gives to life
Will receive what life will give

Day 200

Pass your hand to help
And ye shall be helped
Be no hindrance
And there is no need for defense

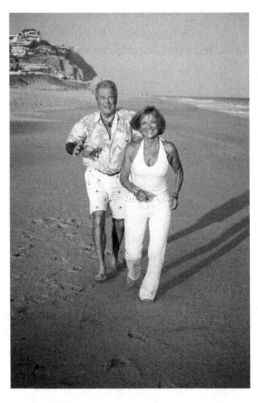

Day 201

Help a friend
Listen and defend
What brings you to a happy end
Before its time to transcend

Day 202

Call me a name
And I shall only pity you
Call me your friend
And you shall need no pity

Day 203

Love and ye shall be happy
Hate and ye shall go unloved
And when it is time to be happy
All past relationships aren't removed

Day 204

Help the needy and ye shall
Be needed; be needed and
Ye shall be loved
(An oxymoron since love is
dependent on need not need dependent on love)

Day 205

Words are hollow when spoken
By a hollow voice
Words are strength when spoken
With conviction to rejoice
The intent and content make sound a token

Day 206

Love as if you'll die tomorrow
Live as if you'll know no sorrow
Build as if you'll live forever
Believe in now rather than never

Day 207

If you haven't loved with abandon
You'll never know
What it's like to be left standing
After she has said no

Day 208

Save my spirit for the days that are black
Have me find the answers that I lack
So when the sun shines and the wind blows
I am the one that knows, why

Day 209

Help me flow and become the tide
That washes mankind before they have died
Simple logic prevails when we cleanse
Our intentions with preventions

Day 210

Life is funny that way
Eyes will open on Judgment Day
But if death isn't meant to stay
The irreverent must have forgotten how to pray

Day 211

If I start my day standing in the rain
It seems as if I spend it being vain
But if I start off with a dream
Things get better than they seem

Day 212

I'm just like a sundial
That loses its smile
As time passes
My thoughts are gone in a while,
But the sun still rises

Day 213

America deserves her greatness
For to be great is to sacrifice mediocrity
For truth and dedication and affluence
And that's the greatness of any nation's heritage
To be forgotten with the purge
for money and influence

Day 214

The security of the mind's belief
Is much more than the reef
It is the shore after the tide
With fear of failure left behind

Day 215

Those stumbling through one more dance
Wait for life to hand them one more chance
And if life hands them gold on a platter
Stumbling along as if it doesn't matter
That they're fumbling what they scatter

Day 216

Though my heart has bled
I want to assume a firm tread
On a path that Jesus said
Would make a righteous bed
Because whatever I have made
Is where I will be laid

Day 217

Some find the raindrops sad
Some thank God, and the crops are glad
But for me, it's the little peace that I have had
Discerning between good and bad

Day 218

Lay here next to me
Hold me to your security
Speak softly, until my fears are gone
And tomorrow emerges from the dawn
Of my insecurity

Day 219

One's thoughts should go beyond today
Founded on what the ordinary man can say
Up, up and away . . . Down, down to stay
Grounded

Day 220

Oh, this wandering spirit
Hold it dear, for it shall wander
In spite of fear
To never never land
Beyond this earthly sphere

Day 221

How lucky can a person be
That is free of body and mind
Needing no motive to be unkind
Or excuses to unwind

Day 222

They say that all life's great men
Bit off more than they could chew
Lord please fill my mouth
Until it comes true

Day 223

Friendship is the feeling
You can't explain
Like feeling rain
And explaining pain

Day 224

Love is feeling needed
And needing to be felt
By another lost soul
Seeking life's goal
Happiness

Day 225

Life is born to end
But lived in peace as a friend
Its time shall be mighty to amend
With a constitution that will lend
To reuniting as the wind

Day 226

The truth of love is not a dream
It is not a shallow stream
It's the very essence of the mortal theme
To procreate and redeem . . . inhumanity

Day 227

I've asked myself, why. Why friends?
The answer came to me.
It's a sign of our need to exist, as we.

Day 228

Thank God for everything
Yesterday, today and what tomorrow will bring
Unless something goes wrong
Then we must change the song we sing

Day 229

Give more of yourself with mirth
Teach others to be stealth
Receive happiness, good health and wealth
For your ephemeral time on earth

Day 230

He who is charitable
Has everlasting life
Friends, peace, happy memories and a loving wife

Day 231

Give me the hands of Peter
To cast my net in the sea of dreams
Just to see what I can catch in my jeans
And alas find memories in the creases of my schemes

Day 232

Give me the legs and shoulders of Atlas
So I can shrug off the burdens of mankind
And carry more than my load
When my load comes to pass

Day 233

Set your sail to the wind
Tack your rudder to a friend
Break out the map
And plot a course to adapt . . . when, as it must, collapse

Day 234

Give me insight to see myself
Give me foresight to see a friend
Give me hindsight to see us both as we are

Day 235

Give me the foresight to be better
Give me hindsight to be no worse
Give me insight to learn from my own verse

Day 236

My love is knowing wherever you go
And whatever you do, nothing matters
As much as you . . . after all these years of marriage
We have chosen to go wherever and whenever together
By grist or feather

Day 237

Love is choosing to sacrifice your soul
For a person not just a goal
But in the meantime fix that hole
In the heart of her lost soul . . . .

Day 238

How stupid can I be
By wasting the day given to me
And the opportunity
Taken from me

Day 239

Live your life so you say;
"Who cares what time it is
When all I've got is today"
When tomorrow may be my life time gone away

Day 240

How would you use today as the end,
If no tomorrow was to transcend?
Would you spend it as my friend,
Or just defend and condescend,
So plans and memories would just end.

Day 241

Every man must lie before
He can appreciate truth
Every man must feel hated before
He can understand love
Unless of course he loves to hate
and it consumes his heart

Day 242

My mind has often said
That God is in a believer's head
And heaven is fear of being dead
While sinners make their own bed
Here on earth . . . . but my heart says it is the spirit
And I should fear it
As it is my bed to make or break.

Day 243

Life has no end
For those who seek and find the source of the wind
And values that do not bend

Day 244

Like day following night
Death is another light
Shining beyond our mortal sight
From a life of daylight, night lights and fright

Day 245

You treat others as you treat yourself
Treat yourself with love and respect
Then love and respect shall be yours
Unto yourself for others you can love

Day 246

A country, a land, a piece of air
Is only as good as the people there
On a whole America has been fair
Until now when Government is on a tear
With terrorism as the fear

Day 247

Give people nothing to live for
And you shall receive nothing
Give people something to die for
And they shall give you everything

Day 248

The best of America, the worst of the country
The land of the free, the land of futility
Only lies in the will and power of you and me

Day 249

Has America reached its peak?
Have the best done their very best?
Are the critics wearing down the achievers?
Will the trustees destroy trust?
Yes and no depending where the dreamers go
And the doers do!

Day 250

War has hardly slowed the passing years
As man has killed in spite of woman's tears
Believing in hereafter to quell the fears
God can't force peace on the Devil's peers

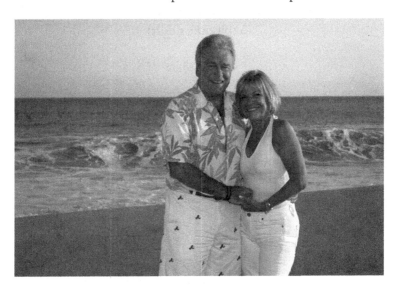

Day 251

If you look, your foe is an open book
Indulge him and you shall see
The friendly side of your former enemy
So, before you advance
Give peace a chance

Day 252

The pursuit of happiness
Is only acclaimed by the pursuer
And distained by the sinner
Which are you? Does any sin fit in your shoe?

Day 253

How lucky can a mortal man be
But to have children as free as he
So heaven can wait while doubters debate
(Who's on the right, who's on the is left
with no one in the middle
to solve the riddle)

Day 254

God giveth, God taketh, God Keepeth
The boundaries of existence
Embrace now as it is given
Embrace hereafter as it is taken
Embrace God so you are not foresaken

Day 255

Love has a double edge
Cutting some and healing
Those who are cut

Day 256

If God is love
Who are you?
The Loved, the lover or the sinner.

Day 257

Dust to Dust
That's the cycle of a fragile leaf
But is it man's reason for grief
Air to Air
That's the cycle of the wind
But is it man's need to comprehend
(That life like leaves and wind, don't end, they just transcend)

Day 258

Forget the pleasure
And forget the lust
Just find someone that you can trust
For their memory not their bust

Day 259

Happiness is what you want
But peace is what you need
And the twain can meet in your heart
While the soul is left to do right

Day 260

Feeling the pleasure of myself
I became insecure
And our love could no longer endure
Then I became unsure
The drama of the impure . . . humanity

Day 261

I' m always looking for something at dawn
I guess it's only fitting to say a prayer
And if it speaks back with sunshine
My life's work will go there

Day 262

Sundown is the closing chapter of this day's life
That finds reality by taking tomorrow as its wife
Hope and charity are married to peace and prosperity
So the future is intact for the people who enact

Day 263

I'm no saint, nor am I pure
But faith is the reason I'm secure
Not taken lightly it will endure

Day 264

Give me enterprise and let me be wise
So progress can escape
Before opportunity dies

Day 265

Enterprise is the sustenance of strife
Don't attack it until you understand it
Then you will want to praise it for sustaining life

Day 266

Doubt is the unwitting stress
Taxing those who don't want less
But it is the energy to outwitting a stressful business

Day 267

Ye are not created equal
We are created to be equal
And in that equation lies
The very birth and girth of our nation

Day 268

I was told as a child
That I never could and I never did
So I've told my children
That never isn't and can forever is
(For that reason that word can't died
A mortal death)

Day 269

Can't died in the arms of the past
While success isn't just not finishing last
It is someone who said "I'll do it now"
Proving never is only as far as learning how

Day 270

Love can grow no higher
Than we can understand
And go no lower than the evil man

Day 271

A bargain always has a sound
Listen and you shall hear
Why lost can be found
If ounces make a pound
And a square meal is put in round

Day 272

Do you want to feel good?
Do you want to feel better?
Do you want to feel needed?
Just tell someone you love them
And allow doubt to go unheeded

Day 273

All of us, only want
To be wanted by our fellow man
To say we are, is to say we can
Love others
A little better than ourselves

Day 274

Hitch your hopes to a star
And go far
Hitch your problems to a stone
And go on alone
To the bottom of Hell's catacomb

Day 275

I hope that you'll pray
Before you hope for peace
And don't get it
For peace is not for hoping but for doing

Day 276

He who prays with purpose and humility
Has admitted he has something to die for
He who lives for humanity
Has everything to live for

Day 277

He who prays will leave a mark,
On those he passes, with charity
If the intent is to be remembered
For wrongs he dismembered

Day 278

A youthful mind is the blood
That makes the oldest heart beat
A youthful heart is the flood
That makes the oldest mind create

Day 279

Sin, lie and bitch, boy
Don't you know it will get you
For the boom-a-rang is no toy
And it will come back to hit you,
Right where that self-righteous boy sits

Day 280

The mind is the grace of God
A gracious mind is the son of God
A mind left behind is given to sin
With a future that's never been

Day 281

Eternal happiness, like a worthy seed,
Isn't what you want, but what you need
What you want is good crops
And a wealth of raindrops

Day 282

Heaven comes to earth
For those who have temporal worth
Good thoughts for the greater good
And no thoughts of should and could

Day 283

Accepting oneself is to admit
That what one needs and what one wants
Are for very different reasons
Like winter, spring, summer and fall seasons

Day 284

Destiny! Is it profound?
Is it a one way road
Or just a dead-end
With futures lost and hopes stowed

Day 285

Plato said of the price of freedom:
All want some
Regardless of need
Until even the dogs demand to intercede

Day 286

The poet is a prophet with words
Of time to come; renewing
Spirits with rhymes to hum
Leaving the cynic deaf and dumb

Day 287

We are what we think we are
To be elsewhere
Is thoughts gone too far
In search of Truth or Dare

Day 288

You don't appreciate getting older
Until fate looks over your shoulder
Then it is time to reconsider
Why we live to wither

Day 289

Success is only a minute away
It just depends on how
You use this minute today
And don't wait for the House and Senate to delay

Day 290

Goodness isn't in the reason why
Just as sight isn't only in an eye
For you see, by your sight
What you think is right
Then goodness can and will prevail

Day 291

Belief can't be yours—Faith shan't be ours
Until you are yours—Until we are ours
And I am yours . . . together we are belief and faith that towers

Day 292

Opportunity is, smiling at adversity
And feeling depression turn to enthusiasm
Missing opportunity is, dwelling in self pity
By letting enthusiasm turn into a prison

Day 293

You can't lose what you haven't got
You can't find what you haven't sought
Nor can happiness be bought
Seek and happiness will get you what you want

Day 294

I built a stairway made of stone
From each day so I'm not alone
Up the stairs to better days
Surrounded by human delays

Day 295

I built a roadway to God's goal
I built a ship for Noah's foal
Hewn from each day so the dock
Became my soul

Day 296

What would the nighttime be
Without the light from eternity
And since it is light years away
It may not exist today, but we do

Day 297

Wings put the future in your hands
Roots sketch your past in the sands
Time will tell of the flight for which it stands

Day 298

Ride the wave and feel the foam
But don't forget to come back home
Because relationships await
At the gates of how beyond the pearly gates of now

Day 299

Raise yourself to positive construction
Don't fall to negative destruction
It is a fine line between war and peace
And a life that will thrive or decease

Day 300

There's still time to believe
In a being that isn't seen
If you believe what you feel
That being is your dream

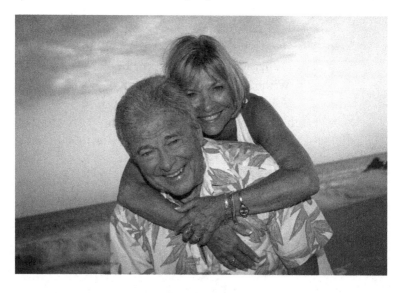

Day 301

Hope is reserved for those
Who see visions of a smoother slope
And take action to cope
Beyond human pain or illegal dope

Day 302

Remember—
In the old days it was important to look good
In these days it's more important to be good
Dress and act like you should
And the todays will be good

Day 303

You measure a life by progress
Not by the years gone by
Take a measure from here to there
And you will have your height, weight and will to care.

Day 304

Progress is great to look
Back upon
It's the risk you took
And Won

Day 305

Humility is the best teacher
But first you must learn
To be humble
And get up from each stumble
As reality starts to crumble

Day 306

Friendship is a means to an end
There's no love without a friend
And love is the beginning and the end

Day 307

Buy a one way ticket to ride
With the love of your life
And nothing to hide
But the pride of having a faithful wife

Day 308

Help is on its way
If you learn to pray, amen
But first you must believe
That thought can inure and relieve sin

Day 309

Righteousness is a word in my song
If I can admit I'm wrong
Self-righteousness is an attitude
That defies sincerity and gratitude

Day 310

It's not what you think
you're worth
That counts
It counts more
If you prove it.

Day 311

Don't knock it
Unless you know you're not jealous
And even then
It may be your turn to be a has been

Day 312

Love as if you'll die tomorrow
In the arms of your lover
But love it today

Day 313

Work as if you'll live forever
But don't forget to thank God for today
And take tomorrow off
To rest not play golf

Day 314

Quell your temptation to frustrate
What was taught in the Psalms?
"As in service you give
And in giving you shall partake"

Day 315

It's good to look upon a dream as real
Expressing what you think and really feel
But don't get too carried away
For a fantasy can't live beyond the break of day

Day 316

Freedom, a bird in flight
A string-less kite, a nocturne at night
Or feeling just right . . . no matter how you look at it
We are free to string our kite, see at night and feel alright

Day 317

If you've never risked your neck
You'll never know
What it's like to find your way
Around a mental wreck

Day 318

If you haven't flown with abandon
You'll never know
What it's like to be a fly without a landin'

Day 319

If God is to finally do us under
Skeptics will finally appreciate
Life and death's full wonder

Day 320

If I start my day off standing in the rain
It seems as if I spend it being vain
But if I start off with a dream
Things get better than they seem

Day 321

Tis the mortal sundial
Left to smile as day time passes
Darkened as human compasses
Have their deeds stand trial

Day 322

All I want to be
Are the thoughts I haven't been lately
And that better person I want to set free

Day 323

The Princess of Wales deserves greatness
For she sacrificed her Aristocracy
To never be called "your highness"
While earning her mark on history
Through alleviating poverty and misery

Day 324

To demand equality
Is to demand immortality
For to demand is a shallow
Threat to act equal
As you die crying, save me!

Day 325

Give me something to work for
And I'll give you everything
Give me nothing to work for
And you can count on nothing

Day 326

I want to wear the same thread
That Jesus said would make a
Righteous bed spread
Before my time is dead

Day 327

Chasing night flight fireflies
Hoping to feel the warmth of burning eyes
Focused on a day dream
Making night sight a sun beam

Day 328

How fortunate can a man be
To have the fortune of being free
With no price on his head
And his value added instead

Day 329

It is said all great men large and small
Bite off more than they can chew
Lord, my mouth is so full
I hope it's really true

Day 330

God giveth, God taketh
If you don't believe
Then try to take it without giving
Live without loving
And you will find Hell in your Kitchen

Day 331

Give me enterprise or give me death
What else is worth each breath
And good intentions And meaningful inventions

Day 332

Those who are enterprising
And create
Contribute the lines to the
Map of fate

Day 333

Now is gone forever
But tomorrow is always there
Lurking behind the urge to dare
And ambitions with a flair

Day 334

Healing the spirit
Is good feelings; don't fear it
Finding the reason
Is good dealings; don't queer it

Day 335

Sing me your song
And I'll tell you what's wrong
Tell me what you see
And I'll sing what you're going to be

Day 336

When your heart opens you will find
Your acts aren't far behind
Along with good deeds you unwind

Day 337

He who waits for the time to come
Awaits for the kingdom
And his will shall become
Happiness, as all is done

Day 338

Do you know
Do you hear
Listen and learn
To be aware
By showing you care

Day 339

Any idiot can be cynical
Only a fool ignores fate
But goodness begets eternal happiness
Come unto me, oh captain of faith

Day 340

Put ink in the historians pen
With a persistent will to define sin
Put eyes in the glasses of kin
So they can study the nature of men . . .
and where we've all been

Day 341

Life is profound competition
Man versus Himself
Who will win and who will be the has been
"The answer my friend is blowing in the wind"

Day 342

Faith that be with you
Is more than doubt beheld against you
Certainty and bold words are cavorting
But positive thoughts are never distorting

Day 343

Let the miserable
Believe themselves happy
For they who seek misery
Have found no destiny

Day 344

He who is charitable
Shall have everlasting wealth, health and be noble;
Not just to stay happy but prone to be able
And grow with each foible

Day 345

Life is but a gamble
Gambling every day
What you're willing to wager
Is what life's willing to pay

Day 346

Look beyond your presence
And find a world
Larger than your own existence
Offering successes and challenges thought foiled

Day 347

Funny how heaven waits
For no one who hesitates
But Hell will freeze over
If you stop and smell the clover

Day 348

Heaven's on earth
Given birth
By the mother
Of a seeking mind
And a father
Of seek and find

Day 349

Hallelujah I'm free
I can see what I want to be
The bad boss made no fool of me
My gut willed his destiny

Day 350

Effort tis the words we say
Of the small man, in a big way
(Ordinary small people
making big extraordinary pay)

Day 351

I believe in those that will
I pity the ones who think they can't
For can't never did anything
And Can did do everything Can't didn't do

Day 352

With no motives, no lies
As within you lives
Ideals; that's the prize;
No surprise that motivation
Is the first step to creation

Day 353

If you hold yourself as true
You'll find a life to please
Never fearing when it's through
Nor giving into a mind's disease

Day 354

Truth is a spell
You can't deceive
Unless you live in earthly hell
With no will to achieve

Day 355

Love is just another word
for Security
If you are secure, you're loved
And when you reject love
You have ruled out immortality

Day 356

Never is just another word
For something you don't want
Or could never find
and should never have sought

Day 357

Happiness is the something
For which the unhappy search
And the loving find
In their every day, boring, mundane life

Day 358

Hardship isn't a test
It's a state of mind
And if you don't mind; tis
The definition of seek and ye shall find

Day 359

Work is each man's expression of himself
Invest a penny and receive no more
Invest a purpose and get far more
An investment for evermore

Day 360

Dreaming is the mental vision
Of man's potential to work
Creativity is putting man's potential in sight
And his abilities to work

Day 361

Infinity is man's explanation
Of what he cannot explain
Or a need to find an EM=C/2 sign
That expresses time

Day 362

The sun is the only sign
Of perfection
In our world
Of reflection
Look upon it
With affection
For it
Shall ever end

Day 363

Don't stir the devil
Unless you can stand a hot handle
And a cold heart

Day 364

Give your children
Roots and wings
Don't tether them
To money and things

Day 365

Smile and ye shall be healed
Heal and ye shall be smiled upon
Warming each day of the year
Making your miracles appear

The prescription has been ordered . . . are you going to take the success pill? Are you fishing for the answer or are you pulling in the dream fish?

Be a Voice to be Heard:
One who accepts today's challenges
Doesn't doubt tomorrow's opportunity
Nor regret yesterday failures
Be life's echo:
The listener's whisper
The speaker's voice
Expressing successes of mankind
And you will be a . . . .

True Success
At Last

SELF-HEALTH ATTAINED

You now are in the Self-Health of life's quantum paradigm determining your life's quality and date of departure to the next continuum . . . by being able to avoid the dangers of the Red Zone you will avoid getting run over by illness . . . living in a Self-Health Zone in route to eternal wellness:

S cience

E ngineered

L ife

F ulfillment

H ow you think determines your life time

E at when you are hungry and stop when you are full determines your weight

A ge is not a factor to measure your longevity

L ife is your show and stage so act on it

T ime is a factor only in your use of it

H ealth is a journey not a destination

Healthy . . . Body . . . Mind . . . Heart . . . Soul = Self Health

Jerry Rhoads

Success
At Last

What is Success
Is it the man who climbs the highest Mountain
Or the woman who swims the widest sea
Or is it the team that somehow wins
Or the person who stands amid fame and fortune
Or is it possible, it's you or me
Let's take a look and see

Are you good at what you do
Do you take pride in living
Are you bright instead of blue
And do you get joy from giving

Are you an open book
With passages to be read
Inviting a passerby's look
Even when you're dead

Will you children be proud to say
"That's my mom and dad,
They helped put me on my way
And taught me good from bad"

If you can honestly say, these things
I feel you certainly can confess
That what your life brings
Is a bountiful success

At Last

By: Jerry L. Rhoads

REFERENCE LIST

The BLUE ZONE: Dan Buettner's Chronicles the "Lessons for Living Longer from the People Who've Lived the Longest published by National Geographic Society 4/21/2009

Jerry Rhoads' Self-Health Series

> *Remedy Eldercide, iUniverse 2009*
> *Restore Elder Pride, iUniverse 2012*
> *Never Too Old to Live, Xlibris 2012*
> *The Boomers Are Coming, Xlibris 2012*

The American Enterprise Party, Xlibris 2013 by Jerry Rhoads

American Enterprise Economics by Jerry Rhoads, CPA

Obama Care, "Affordable Healthcare Act"

The American Enterprise Manifesto, Xlibris 2013

Freakonomics and *Super Freakonomics*, by Steven Levitt and Stephen Dubner

THE RED ZONE DOWNSIZER

With the average weight of Americans, at all ages in the Red Zone, escalating at a troublesome rate we must formulate solutions that move individuals to their ideal BMI. The author's "Downsizer Formula" is a failsafe tool to direct the reduction of weight by increasing physical activity for mental fitness.

Weights by category:

> More than two-thirds (68.8 percent) of adults are considered to be overweight or obese.
> More than one-third (35.7 percent) of adults are considered to be obese.
> More than 1 in 20 (6.3 percent) have extreme obesity.
> Almost 3 in 4 men (74 percent) are considered to be overweight or obese.
> The prevalence of obesity is similar for both men and women (about 36 percent).
> About 8 percent of women are considered to have extreme obesity.

Obesity is predicted to be the highest cause of premature death, chronic disease and over utilization of health care services. Obesity is considered to be a disease of the mind rather than the body. To help those that decide to become what they want to be I have developed the downsizer formula tied to exercise processes that each individual can choose and plan their weight reduction and attainment of their desired BMI.

END NOTES (AUTHOR'S OPINIONS)

1) Premise that America's health is transferable as a culture not as an individual transformation is false.
2) Culturally America is in the Red Zone of health due to poor life style habits.
3) To move America from the Red Zone to the Blue Zone takes a change in American's thinking not changes in their environment or the influence of other dissimilar cultures.
4) Obama Care will lead us further down the path that grandiose Government intervention shall change American values and eventually its collective health.
5) The true solution is to change the Red Zone thinking using economic incentives to attain the individual's moral incentive of better health and a better, longer life…for example tax deductions for wellness expenditures and elimination of harmful chemicals being ingested at an ever increasing rate. Kill the pills and save the wills of Americans.
6) The self-health approach puts the cost of poor health habits squarely in the laps of the offenders and as with any other bad habit the expensive responsibility for paying for them.

ABOUT THE AUTHOR

Jerry Rhoads is a CPA and a Fellow in the American College of Health Care Administrators. He has written three books on health care operations and three books on Self-Health care processes and more than 100 published magazine articles on health care reimbursement and cost systems topics.

He is currently president and chief executive officer of All-American Care Centers, Caregiver Management Systems Inc., a management consulting and software firm specializing in long-term care. He created the caregiver charting, staffing, and cost system while running two skilled nursing facilities and a CCRC.

He wrote the white paper in 1975 on case-mix reimbursement for HCFA that led to MDS and RUGs development. He also sat on the HEW and HHS committees in the 1970s and 1980s that formulated the current RAI linkage to case-mix formulas based on nursing minutes of care.

Jerry was president and chief executive officer of his own CPA firm that began in 1977 and grew into a consulting firm and software development company. Prior to that, he was a partner in two other CPA firms after leaving the Health Care Consulting Division of Arthur Andersen & Co. in 1969. While there, he was assigned to head up the Blue Cross of America project for auditing claims and cost reports as the first fiscal intermediary for the entire country when Medicare and Medicaid legislation was originally passed and implemented. He later was the partner in charge of the Aetna Insurance Company Fiscal Intermediary project for auditing claims and cost reports.

Over the years Jerry has written extensively on his specialty Health Care. Now that Obama Care has passed and is bearing down on small business he is on a campaign to shift the paradigm away from Government run health care to an Enterprise Model where SHIFT means **S**elf-**H**ealth **I**nsurance **F**unding **T**rust. This is where the individuals are responsible for setting up their own withholding trust account with a Mutual Health Insurance Company and deciding how to spend their own money on prevention, wellness programs, preserving social, relationships and mental health, with treatment as the last resort. It eliminates $600 billion in waste in the current punitive regulatory system and takes the bureaucrats out of the middle of making decisions on each American's money and how it is spent on health and fitness leading to personal wellness.

JERRY'S WAR STORIES

Jerry Rhoads as a Son

George and Velma Rhoads were my parents. Born in Missouri during the Depression years, they worked all their lives for a comfortable retirement that never came. They were neither particularly healthy nor wealthy. In their later years, chronic maladies took their toll.

George had worked in the factory at Firestone and contacted respiratory problems from asbestos. He had looked forward to being sixty-four so he could get away from the drudgery of work. At the age of eighty-two, he died in a nursing home where he had been for the better part of four years. Prior to going to the nursing home, he had a stroke that impaired his functioning somewhat but it was the respiratory problems that prevailed. During the time he was in the nursing home, he fractured his ankle and his wrist due to staff-related accidents. At the latter stages of the emphysema, he was put on continuous oxygen. This was the beginning of the end due to his dependence on a certain saturation rate during the night he was delirious and was given sedatives to quiet him. Not only was the protocol harmful, but eventually killed him. At no time did a doctor see him more often than every ninety days. During that time, he received on average five telephone orders for lab tests, medications, and other doctor-ordered tests that led to furthering his demise.

Velma, my mother, had heart problems related to blood thinners that were prescribed for her as she aged. But the real problem was her digestive system. Diverticulitis developed and she had to have a portion of her colon removed and a colostomy inserted. Having been on blood thinners prior to the operation, she had a blood clot during surgery and stroked. From that point on, she could not walk, talk nor move her right side. Her mind was still there but she could not communicate. She followed my father in death at the age of eighty-four, at the same nursing home as a vegetable. To stop the suffering, she was taken off life support and starved to death over a ten-day period.

On numerous occasions, I voiced concern and unhappiness about the lack of staff and the misuse of my father and mother's Medicare benefits. The care was subpar, there was never any staff available on the weekends, and it was inevitable that their passing would be inhumane.

Jerry Rhoads' Initiatives as an Administrator

At Fox Valley Nursing Center, in Elgin, Illinois and Carington Living Center in Glendale Heights, Illinois we set up restorative and psycho/social programs for improving the patients functioning through the following activities:

- o Bowling league using plastic pins and balls
- o Fitness trail for exercise
- o Resistance training using light weights and pulleys
- o Gourmet club on Saturday and Sunday nights
- o Sewing club for sale at the annual Bazaar
- o Knitting club for sale at the annual Bazaar
- o Card club
- o Current events club
- o Personal history club
- o Newcomers club
- o Stroke club

- o Respiratory club
- o Heart and soul club
- o Theater club and karaoke time
- o Happy hour

We also had the more functional patients sorting and folding clothes for which they were paid. All females had their hair done once a week and the men once a month. We had a security plan that includes a functional patient checking locked doors at night. We had an Ambassador Club that met every Friday for voicing problems that needed to be addressed the next week. A member of the staff participated along with the resident representative, a family member, the administrator, and a volunteer.

The most memorable people that helped me pull facilities out of the gutter were at Carington. Wally was an ambulatory patient that wanted to be helpful and Irene was the Resident Council President that wanted to improve the conditions. Both became my friends and helpers in keeping an eye out for problems and being my eyes and ears during the weekends and nights. They were the reporters to the Ambassador's Club that fixed physical and staff problems as they were occurring. Initially they were called Jerry's spies, then they became my ambassadors of goodwill and care. Both of these soldiers of fortune died after I left Carington, probably of a broken heart because I gave them hope and a purpose and the successors gave them a warehouse again.

At Fox Valley, a 207-bed skilled nursing facility, in 1987 the problems manifested themselves in staffing. The staff morale was low and resulted in no shows and walk-offs. The state surveyors called it Death Valley because of the problems from the past. One Sunday, I received a call at home that the surveyors entered the center at midnight for the stated purpose of doing a focused review of the care and staffing. I personally drove to the nurse aides' houses to pick them up to work that night shift or we would have been closed. One CNA voiced concern because she had been drinking all day. I had no choice but bring her in and ask her to stay out of the way of the surveyors. Fortunately, I was able to satisfy them with my commitment to make changes immediately. It was shortly thereafter that the infamous snow storm happened and half the staff came together as teams and ran the place better for three days. From that point on, the staff organized the care in teams and met the patient's needs consistently, and we were awarded the five stars of quality in our next survey. When the facility was sold in 1989 it had 195 patients, thirty-four Medicare cases and was generating over $3.5 million per year in revenue. Prior to the turn-a-round the census was 167 with four Medicare cases and $2 million in revenue.

Interestingly, when I got to Fox Valley, then Carington, the staff did not know what the state's quality incentive payment was all about. Quip as it was called paid a bonus of $2 per patient per day if you scored on all of their six criteria of quality. The criteria were called stars and focused on environment, care planning, family involvement, patient satisfaction, productive activities, and infection control. So we went from the staff not knowing what a star was to earning all of them in a matter of days at Fox and a matter of weeks at Carington. How is this possible? Well, we went from departments to teams, we went from warehousing to care housing, and the end result was better care at a lower cost: turnover was reduced from 200% to less than 20%, unapproved absenteeism went away and the disregard for the patients' needs dissolved overnight. More revenue less cost better care what a formula.

At Carington, in 1989, the staff was again initially resistant to change but responded to the plan to focus their time on the patients' needs with time to socialize with the patients as well as prioritize their care. We were initially rejected for certification by the VA due to lack of programming, but later on a follow-up visit they could not believe the number of programs we had going daily. At that point the social service staff was conducting thirteen psycho/social programs daily along with rehab nursing and restorative care being provided to those that needed it on a daily basis. It was their opinion that we were better than the flagship called White Hall. Of course, we got their certification and backing. When I got to Carington, the census was 175 out of 206 beds, they had four Medicare patients and the revenue was around $2.5 million. Twenty-two months later, we had 197 patients with an average Medicare caseload of fifty-five and annualized revenue of $5 million. Not only did we have the highest Medicaid rate in the state, but we had convinced Medicare to raise the daily rate by $75 per day for rehabbing and restoring cases back home.

Jerry Rhoads' Initiatives as a Consultant

In 1979 at the Methodist Retirement Center in Lawrenceville, Illinois, there was no active Medicare program and the old shelter care building was slated for demolition. I was brought in as a consultant to help the board avoid bankruptcy. We proceeded to devise an action plan that would raise $3 million in tax-exempt bonds for restoring the shelter care building into an assisted-living concept. Thirty beds were certified for Medicare and a new Administrator hired to run the business affairs replacing a Methodist Preacher who had let the operation go downhill. Today, the Continuing Care concept that was implemented twenty-five years ago is the flagship for long-term care services in Southern Illinois. They have added duplexes, condos, and townhouses for the elderly.

In 2003, Christian Homes (an eleven-nursing home chain in Missouri and Arkansas) engaged my firm to capture the Medicare billings that were justified by the use of the Caregiver Management System utilizing the regulatory requirements of Fox v Bowen and Transmittal 262. Unbeknownst to that organization, they had been incorrectly instructed by their intermediary that they could not bill for anything except certain procedures specified by the interpretations of CMS (the paying agency for Medicare). Once we got involved in mapping out the care that Medicare was to pay for and supported their billing with this documentation, the revenue streams increased an average of 30% per facility. Since the state Medicaid programs were cutting back, this represented and instant life support correction for all of their facilities. To date, the system has justified upward to $8 million more in annual billings less the savings to the Medicaid program of $4 million.

In 2002, Nursing Home Managers (a five-nursing home chain in Illinois) engaged my firm to capture lost Medicare billings. Over a three year period that group was able to stop sending bills to the state of Illinois Medicaid program and generate another $5 million in revenue.

In 2004, we were engaged by Pinnacle health Care (with thirteen homes in Arkansas and Missouri) to do the same thing and generated over $11 million per year in additional Medicare billings.

In 2004, we were engaged by ABCM Corporation (operator of thirty-one nursing homes in Iowa) to assist them in capturing lost Medicare revenue. To date, they have implemented Caregiver Management System in six of their homes and have successfully improved their Medicare performance by 25%.

In 2003, were engaged by HMR Corporation (operator of twenty-five nursing homes in South Carolina) to assisted them in capturing lost Medicare revenue in two of their homes.

In 2006, we were engaged by an owner of two skilled nursing facilities in Iowa. They were in financial difficulty and did not think they could afford us. We finally got ABCM to recommend us and to date, both have implemented Caregiver Management Systems. In the one home they had no Medicare cases and in thirty days improved to fifteen active cases. In the other facility, they went from four to eight the first day of training by bringing patients back on Medicare that had been inappropriately discontinued. At this rate, the two homes will produce $2.3 million more in revenue and can be solvent.

Over the last fifteen years we have put the system in over 140 facilities in twenty-two different states (a chain in Utah of fourteen, a chain of eleven in Texas, New Mexico, Louisiana and Oklahoma, a chain of ten in Ohio, a chain of three in Arizona, a not-for—profit group of six CCRCs in Ohio, homes in Nebraska, New York, California, Indiana, thirty-three facilities in Illinois, a chain of eleven in Missouri, a chain of thirteen in Arkansas etc.) that generated over $150 million in annual Medicare revenue while saving Medicaid $50 million per year. This has resulted in more patients being restored and going home. In that period of time over 40,000 more patients have been discharged home than before. Not only does it improve the quality, it enables the nursing homes to fix the building, the parking lots, provide better working conditions to the staff which improves morale, and lowers turnover and absenteeism. It truly is a win-win situation.

Jerry Rhoads' Paradigm Shift

In 1987 while running Fox Valley Rehabilitation Center I was sent the classic court case that would change my career and life.

Fox v Bowen and Transmittal 262 (Connecticut 1986); then Jimmo v Sebelius was issued October 26, 2012 (Vermont 2012)—Federal judges issued opinions that find the Federal Government in violation of Title XVIII of the Social Security Act depriving the elderly, disabled and infirm of their rightful Medicare benefits.

Where does the federal government stand on what we are doing? Is it gaming the system or committing fraud and abuse of the Medicare program? I was notified by Aetna Insurance company that a court case had been issued in 1986 that would enable me to hold the Social Security Administration and the Department of

Health and Human Services accountable to the Medicare insurance policy and what constitutes the obligation of Medicaid as the last resort for payment for nursing homes.

The use of Fox v Bowen and Transmittal 262 as the basis for providing the skilled services and documenting the physician and nurse involvement in the daily care the government must pay by law. Most providers and consultants are not schooled in this nor do they know how to plan the care, deliver the care, and defend the claims. As a result, typically the nursing homes are afraid to send the bill and opt to bill private resources then Medicaid instead. Since Medicare is the only pay source that pays for truly restoring the patients they end up on welfare for the rest of their lives. This way, the facility loses money, the family loses their loved one, the patient loses hope, and the state Medicaid programs end up with bills they should not be paying.

For example, our client in Arkansas has Blue Cross of Arkansas as the fiscal intermediary. As we helped their thirteen facilities stop billing Medicaid inappropriately and billing Medicare, justifiably Blue Cross stopped payment on over 200 claims amounting to over $2 million. This was done in violation of Fox v Bowen and Transmittal 262. An attorney for the provider brought this to Blue Cross' attorney who advised the intermediary to pay the claims. Prior to that, we had appealed thirty-seven cases to the administrative law judges and won all of them. So in effect, the government was illegally withholding funds from the providers. We were not afraid to confront them and eventually prevailed. Over the last twenty years, my firm has done this a number of times where majority of the providers acquiesce and do not establish a claim. If and when the problem gets fixed nationally, most of the providers will be left out in the cold with Medicaid on their heels.

Why hasn't this problem been fixed? It will eventually when the masses realize that we have to restore the elderly, not just warehouse them in nursing homes. (as predicted by this statement the Center of Medicare Advocacy sued CMS for misapplying the Medicare entitlement to Part A coverage by challenging the use of Improvement Standard as a rule of thumb used for the purpose of denying entitled coverage to Medicare beneficiaries, bringing an end to Medicare's long-practiced but illegal application of an "Improvement Standard." The settlement of the case [Jimmo v. Sebelius, No. 5:11-cv-00017 (D.Vt.)] will improve access for tens of thousands of Americans, especially older adults and people with disabilities, whose Medicare coverage is denied or terminated because these beneficiaries are considered "not improving" or "stable." Resolution of this legal challenge effectively ends this harmful practice and ensures fair coverage rules for those who live with chronic conditions and rely on Medicare to cover basic, necessary health care.

> : "Medicare should cover essential care for the treatment and management of chronic conditions. This Settlement offers a real opportunity to finally eliminate the use of the unfair Improvement Standard to deny these claims."

> Lead plaintiff Glenda Jimmo is a 76 year old resident of Bristol, Vermont. Blind since the age of nineteen, she is confined to a wheelchair as a result of her disabling conditions, including a below-the-knee amputation. She requires regular skilled nursing services in her home to provide wound care and help manage her condition. She is proud to have had the opportunity to challenge this illegal Medicare policy, and relieved to know that her care, and the care for thousands of other older people and people with serious disabilities, will be covered by Medicare.

> "Filing the Settlement agreement begins a long process to reverse the damage done to tens of thousands of Medicare beneficiaries with chronic conditions,"

Jerry Rhoads

observed plaintiffs' lead counsel Gill Deford. The court's tentative approval of the Settlement will be followed by notification to the class members, who will have an opportunity to comment in writing and at a hearing on the proposed settlement, after which the judge will make her final decision on the Settlement.

Under the proposed Settlement, a nationwide class of beneficiaries will be certified, numerous parts of the Medicare Benefit Policy Manual will be rewritten, and CMS will carry out an educational campaign for providers, Medicare contractors and adjudicators. The revised CMS manual language will clarify that Medicare coverage is available for maintenance services when skilled personnel are required to perform or supervise the care or therapy safely and effectively. In addition, many class members will have an opportunity to have their previously denied claims reviewed under the revised Medicare standards. Plaintiffs' attorneys will monitor and, if necessary, enforce the provisions of the agreement.

While the Centers for Medicare & Medicaid Services (CMS), which is the federal agency responsible for the Medicare program, continues to deny the existence of the rule of thumb known as the "Improvement Standard," beneficiaries and advocates know that contractors and other adjudicators repeatedly rely on it to deny Medicare claims. Nationwide, thousands of cases of the illegal and unjust practice were identified in 2011 alone.

The lawsuit was brought in United States District Court in Burlington, Vermont by seven individual plaintiffs from Vermont, Connecticut, Rhode Island, Maine and Pennsylvania and seven national organizational plaintiffs: the National Committee to Preserve Social Security and Medicare, the National Multiple Sclerosis Society, Parkinson's Action Network, Paralyzed Veterans of America, the American Academy of Physical Medicine and Rehabilitation, the United Cerebral Palsy Association and the Alzheimer's Association. The plaintiffs joined with the named defendant, Secretary of Health and Human Services Kathleen Sebelius, in asking the federal judge to approve the settlement of the case on October 16, 2012.

Jerry Rhoads' Major Accomplishment:

- A Wonderful marriage for 54 years to the same high school sweetheart Sharon Kay White Rhoads
- Four wonderful, happy, healthy and prosperous children: Christie Caye Stephens, Kimber Leigh Lawrence, Kip Alan Rhoads, Kelli Jo Ahern
- Twelve wonderful, happy, healthy and prosperous grand children: Alex, Chad, Leigh Stephens, Blake, Derek, Paris Lawrence, Celena, Fallon, Tyler, Nicholas, Rhoads, Nathan, Troy Ahern
- One great grandson, to date, who will be happy, healthy and prosperous: Carter Michael Stephens.
- Started 10 small businesses from a CPA firm to a management consulting company, to a software company, a publishing company, a reimbursement consulting business, a nursing home management company, a co-owner of two skilled nursing facilities and a real estate investment LLC. Over the years employed hundreds of people in these businesses.
- A Possible run for Governor of Iowa in 2014 and President in 2016 as the candidate for the American Enterprise Party that I formed to promote my ideas on self-health and self-preservation in the "former land of the free".

Jerry Rhoads

IF YOU HAVE READ THIS FAR I COMMEND YOU FOR BEING POSITIVE AND ACTION ORIENTED USING YOUR MOST VALUABLE ASSET . . . YOUR MIND. I ALSO CONGRATULATE, IF YOU CHOOSE, FOR ENDING RED ZONE THINKING AND HABITS TO PURSUING THE END ZONE OF BETTER HEALTH HABITS AND LIFE STYLE. JERRY RHOAD, AUTHOR

For information on the American Enterprise Party look up my other books on Amazon's Kindle network or go to www. americanenterpriseparty.com

For information on change in lifestyle fitness based on input efforts for measurable outcome results go to www.americaintheredzone.com and utilize the DOWNSIZER algorithms for determining BMI, calorie burn for weight loss over periods of time, and improvement in BMI in a real time mode. The Self-Health formula is simple . . . calorie burn times repetition equals weight loss and Self-Image gains. Leading aspiring Americans out of the Red Zone life style into the Self-Health end zone thus creating a Blue Zone culture.